How to Ship Sperm on the Internet: Get Pregnant Without Ever Having Sex, Paying a Sperm Bank, or Leaving Your Home

By Joe Donor

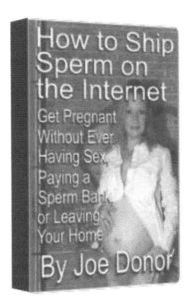

Createspace Edition

Copyright © 2013 Joe Donor.

Acknowledgements

Thanks to Todd Donor, Mike Donor, Eric Donor, Colin Donor, Jens Nergaard, all the baby mommas, others too numerous to mention who made this book possible.

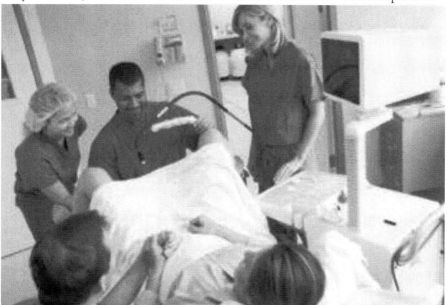

VISIT US ON THE WEB:

Join our Facebook group to find a free donor or become a donor:

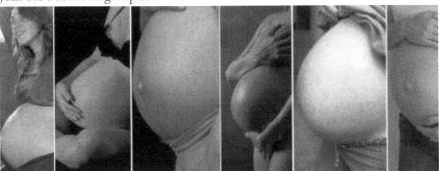

https://www.facebook.com/groups/joesdonorgroup/

Email Joe Donor with questions:
joe00donor@gmail.com

Visit us here for a printed version of this book:
https://www.createspace.com/4714292

Click here to see a YouTube video about this book and other donor topics:
http://youtu.be/-beW8hC3r1o

Click here for other ebooks by Joe Donor on Smashwords:
https://www.smashwords.com/profile/view/joe00donor

Click here for other ebooks by Joe Donor on Amazon USA:
http://www.amazon.com/Joe-Donor/e/B00J59W7BW

Praise for the author from readers

"I appreciate the ease of reading and understanding this guide. I had a few questions about timing insemination at first but once I read this guide ALL my questions and uncertainties were answered. I believe this will help many women who have any questions regarding trying to conceive with an online donor. The pictures were helpful as well; they give more understanding on everything."

In easy to understand language, the author has written a concise guide for both recipients and donors alike interested in either donating or receiving private sperm donations. The author cuts through a lot of technical language, in such a way that the average person can understand private sperm donating to the point where they can easily receive samples and do it in their own private area, safely, and to their own optimal benefit to become pregnant.

A fascinating book, with detailed insemination techniques, how to select donors, what type of questions to ask, how to protect anonymity and the like. With ever-growing interest in private sperm donating, this book written by an experienced sperm donor, offers many valuable tips to help facilitate a safe and optimal chance at getting pregnant.

A must have book for those interested in private sperm donating and receiving!

Joe Donor's previous book "Get pregnant for free on the internet with a private sperm donor without having sex or paying $$$ to a sperm bank" was featured in the Italian magazine Vanity Fair

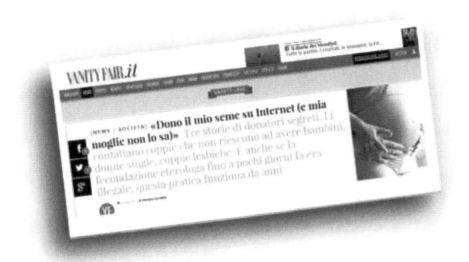

(http://www.vanityfair.it/news/societ%C3%A0/14/04/22/fecondazione-eterologa-storie)

Joe Donor, author of this book, was interviewed in the Italian magazine L'Espresso:

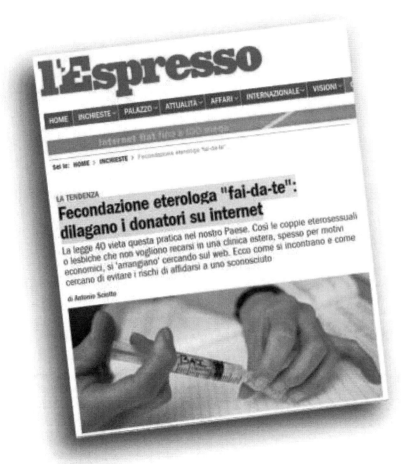

(http://espresso.repubblica.it/inchieste/2013/11/28/news/fecondazione-eterologa-dilaga-il-fai-da-te-1.143296)

Legal information and disclaimer

We are not doctors or lawyers, you are fully responsible for any health, financial, or legal consequences of using an internet sperm donor. Methods discussed here are not the product of scientific research: this is just a layman's discussion of one chilled semen shipping method. Sperm banks freeze and quarantine sperm six months until they can retest the donor to insure his HIV status at time the sperm was collected. This is the gold standard. Since we use chilled not frozen, we cannot insure HIV free status this way, and if you cannot tolerate this risk, you should use a sperm bank. However, most people in the USA get pregnant at home without using a bank or benefiting from bank protections, so we do not feel the health risk of using an internet donor is any worse than the risk those people encounter when conceiving children outside the clinic in conventional family settings. Pregnant women face much more certain and severe medical risk during childbirth than they ever will during conception.

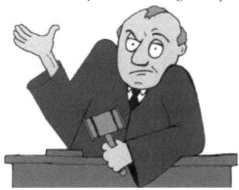

Table of Contents

Acknowledgements	2
VISIT US ON THE WEB:	3
Joe Donor's previous book "Get pregnant for free on the internet with a private sperm donor without having sex or paying $$$ to a sperm bank" was featured in the Italian magazine Vanity Fair	5
Joe Donor, author of this book, was interviewed in the Italian magazine L'Espresso:	6
Legal information and disclaimer	7
TABLE OF CONTENTS	**8**
CHAPTER 1: EFFICACY OF SHIPPING CHILLED SEMEN	**15**
CHAPTER 2: WHAT CAN A RECIPIENT DO TO INCREASE HER CHANCES?	**17**
CHAPTER 3: SHIPPING CHILLED SEMEN: AN ALTERNATIVE TO SPERM BANKS	**19**
Women living in rural areas may have few or no local banks	20
Recipients may have to undergo exams at sperm banks	21
Some banks may even refuse to help single or gay women.	22
Why pay so much more for unnecessary poking and prodding?	23
Banks offer airtight legal protection (at a price), but do you need it?	24
Does the legal protection offered by a bank justify the cost?	25
Private donors offer greater selection	26
CHAPTER 4: HOW CAN I PROTECT MY PRIVACY?	**27**
Will my donor know my home address?	28

Do you want semen delivered here?	29
Always have UPS leave the package without signature	30
No UPS box, no problem	31
What about my Facebook identity?	32
What about my phone number?	33
Chapter 5: How to time your insemination	34
What is an OPK? What is the LH surge?	35
What should I do if I get two positives on the OPK in the same cycle?	36
Timing of typical cycle events	37
Use paper calendar not computer program	38
Cd1 never same day two months in a row	39
Practical example	40
CHAPTER 6: THE OPK (OVULATION PREDICTION KIT)	**41**
Reading test results on the OPK	42
CHAPTER 7: USING BASAL TEMPERATURES TO PREDICT OVULATION	**45**
CHAPTER 8: PREDICT OVULATION FROM CHANGE IN THE CERVIX	**47**
CHAPTER 9: PREDICTING OVULATION WITH MITTELSCHMERZ AND OTHER WAYS	**49**
Other ways to predict ovulation	50
CHAPTER 10: SUMMARY OF KEY CYCLE DATES	**51**
CHAPTER 11: TYB, SHIPPING KITS, AND COLLECTING AND SHIPPING SEMEN	**52**

Cold packs	53
Other cold pack manufacturers	54
What do the recipients do with the parts of the kit after they inseminate?	55
Specimen cup	56
Sperm-Friendly Lubricant	56
The sample, when collected, is coagulated	57
What Does Normal Volume Look Like?	57
You may also collect with a Ziploc bag	58
CHAPTER 12: THE SEMEN EXTENDER	**59**
The manufacturer's directions for using Irvine TYB	60
Open the TYB vial's metal lid using a knife	62
To mix semen and extender more thoroughly, use a pipette	62
After thoroughly mixing the semen with the extender (TYB), transfer the mixture to one or more transport tubes.	63
Water kills semen. Soap residue also kills semen.	63
CHAPTER 13: ALTERNATIVE TO TYB: AN EXTENDER MADE FROM POWDER	**64**
Prepare the powder extender	65
Prepare the powder extender	65
Cut open the small foil envelope containing the powder	66
Dump the powder extender in to the container with the mixing solution.	67
You can also pour the powder directly in to the mixing solution bottle	68
Shake the bottle in order to completely dissolve the powder in the mixing solution	68

To mix semen and extender more thoroughly, use a pipette	69
Sometimes the extender comes in a 10ml amount, with a bottle with 10ml of mixing solution and an envelope with enough powder for 10ml of extender.	70
To divide extender powder in to 5ml portions before you mix the powder and mixing solution:	71
Keep the unused half of the powder in a small, sealed container in a cool, dry place	72
To divide after you mix the powder and mixing solution:	73

CHAPTER 14: OTHER CONTENTS OF THE KIT: THE TRANSPORT VIALS   74

Two 5-ml vials may not be enough	74
Sterile pipettes	75
Insulated foil envelopes	75
You can cut the insulated envelope in half if it is too large	76
Place the vials of extended semen in the insulated envelope	76
Close the envelope and tape it up with duct tape	77
Individually wrapped sterile 10ml syringe	77
Instead Softcup	78
Styrofoam cooler	78
Tape the cooler shut	80
Shipping carton	80

CHAPTER 15: SOLUTIONS FOR DONORS WHO DON'T HAVE ACCESS TO A FREEZER OR SOMEWHERE TO STORE SUPPLIES   81

CHAPTER 16: HOW TO MAKE A HOMEMADE STYROFOAM COOLER   82

A soldering gun is useful to cut Styrofoam	83
When attaching the blade, be sure that it is aligned with the gun barrel	84

Attach the Styrofoam blade to the soldering gun	85
Heat the gun	86
Modify cooler bought in store	87
Measure before cutting	88
Cut with soldering iron	89
Modify the cardboard box	90
Measure cardboard box and cut	91
Homemade shipping kit from modified cardboard box and Styrofoam cooler	92
CHAPTER 17: SHIPPING CHILLED SEMEN IN A THERMOS	**93**
Where to find ready-made coolant?	93
"Reusable ice substitute" as a coolant	94
Consider the shape of the coolant when freezing	94
Be sure to consider weather conditions.	95
CHAPTER 18: DROP OFF AT EXPRESS MAIL COMPANY	**96**
Friday Shipment	97
Insure you paid for Saturday delivery and the label has a Saturday code	98
What if the OPK turns positive on a weekend?	99
Saturday OPK	100
Sunday OPK	101
Benefits of holding packages at The UPS Store, other UPS tips	102
Benefits of holding packages at the express mail company's office and other tips	103
UPS Customer Centers	104

Express mail companies may ask for ID — 105

Drop off boxes — 106

Early morning delivery — 106

CHAPTER 19: FOR RECIPIENTS: BASIC INSEMINATION WITH SYRINGE — 107

Macroscopic examination of the semen (how the semen should appear to the naked eye) — 108

For some reason many women expect more volume — 109

Sterile, individually wrapped, 10ml syringe — 110

If vial mouth is too small, pour semen in cup — 111

Insemination with 10ml syringe (needle-less) — 112

CHAPTER 20: INSEMINATION USING SPECULUM AND CATHETER — 113

Catheter detail — 114

CHAPTER 21: INSTEAD SOFTCUP INSEMINATION — 115

How to insert the Softcup — 116

CHAPTER 22: WHAT ABOUT THE TURKEY BASTER? — 117

The turkey is a large bird that is traditionally eaten on some holidays in the U.S. — 118

The turkey baster is clumsy to use in comparison with a 10ml syringe — 118

CHAPTER 23: CHECK SHIPPED SPERM MICROSCOPICALLY TO SEE IF STILL ALIVE — 119

Micra Hand-held scope specifically for the evaluation of sperm — 120

Prepare a semen smear slide — 121

Use a donor who knows how to evaluate sperm microscopically — 122

CHAPTER 24: WHEN CAN I DO THE HPT (HOME PREGNANCY TEST)?   123

Unusual pregnancy test results   124

A faint test line is a positive on the HPT   125

CHAPTER 25: HOW FAR AWAY CAN I SHIP?   126

However, even though technology improves, new legal restrictions cause delays.   127

International shipping from Germany to France and from Germany to the UK   128

Shipping from the USA to Scotland?   129

CHAPTER 26: USE A CHEMICAL HEATING AND COOLING PACK TO PREVENT FREEZING IN EXTREME COLD   130

CHAPTER 27: TESTING A PROTOTYPE OF SHIPPING KIT   131

OTHER BOOKS BY JOE DONOR   132

"Get Pregnant For Free on the Internet With a Private Sperm Donor Without Having Sex or Paying $$$ to a Sperm Bank"   132

"True Stories of Pregnancy by PI, or Partial Intercourse, With Free Sperm Donors"   133

Chapter 1: Efficacy of Shipping Chilled Semen

Many women ask: "What are my chances?"

As a donor with many first cycle successes, I know that I am offering that possibility from my side, I think a woman's chances with me are as good as they would be with anyone else, but that is not to say every woman will succeed in the first cycle. Much depends on her underlying fertility, age, health, and lifestyle. Much also depends on luck. Although there are no studies available in humans, we know from studies in animal breeding that chilled semen is about half as effective as fresh semen (i.e., such as sexual intercourse) and about twice as effective as frozen semen. If we assume that pregnancy occurs in about 20% of cycles in which fertile women have sexual intercourse with a fertile male during the most fertile time of their cycles (this is a widely accepted figure), and that chilled shipped semen is about half as effective, then the expected percentage of women who fall pregnant during or before each successive cycle in which they inseminate with chilled shipped semen, in comparison with the expected percentage of women who fall pregnant by sexual intercourse, would look something like this:

Cycle	1	2	3	4	5	6
Shipping	10.0%	19.0%	27.1%	34.4%	41.0%	46.9%
Fresh	20.0%	36.0%	48.8%	59.0%	67.2%	73.8%

Cycle	7	8	9	10	11	12
Shipping	52.2%	57.0%	61.3%	65.1%	68.6%	71.8%
Fresh	79.0%	83.2%	86.6%	89.3%	91.4%	93.1%

By way of comparison, in "Clinical Methods: The History, Physical, and Laboratory Examinations," a 1990 text book, authors Hatcher & Kowal cite an unwanted pregnancy rate of 89%: out of 100 women who started out the year not wanting to become pregnant but also not taking any action to prevent pregnancy. It is very close to the 93.1% we would expect to get pregnant within a year of trying to conceive.

My success rate, 4 positive pregnancy tests after about 30 cycles of shipping reflects a 1st cycle success rate, as most women quit after 1-2 cycles, and many who try longer are older or heavier. Statistically, a few women will get pregnant in the first cycle, but many won't. The women who don't succeed right away often become discouraged and give up.

Unfortunately many women who want to work with a free donor may suffer from diabetes, polycystic ovary syndrome (pcos), advanced maternal age, tobacco dependency, etc., and aren't in the healthiest, most fertile category of women who would expect to fall pregnant in 20% of cycles in which they try to conceive with fresh semen.

If for example they were half as fertile as the most fertile women, expecting to get pregnant in 10% of cycles with fresh semen, then those women wouldn't be hitting the 50% success threshold until around one year of trying.

So, women who want to become pregnant using shipped semen would want to plan on six months of trying if they are a healthy, height-weight-proportional 20-year-old and maybe plan on 12 months of trying if they are obese, a heavy smoker, or 40+ years old.

If you're reading this and you're overweight, don't envy thin women just yet. I've known more than one very fit recipient who had difficulty getting pregnant which I suspect was caused by low body fat due to a very strict physical fitness regimen. I have also known women to experience difficulty getting pregnant and issues during pregnancy due to rapid weight loss on a fad diet. Moderation in all things is the key. I recommend try to walk 30 minutes a day, and stop drinking all beverages except for water, as a way to moderately reduce weight. Trying to conceive while overweight may ultimately be better than waiting to lose weight, or embarking on an extreme diet/exercise program. Just understand it may take longer than the average.

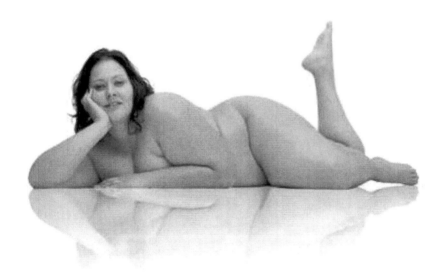

Chapter 2: What can a recipient do to increase her chances?

I don't know of any herb, vitamin, or other therapy that will make a woman more fertile. Yes, there are "prenatal" vitamins; folic acid is often recommended for women who are trying to conceive. However, those are to make a woman's body more hospitable for the pregnancy, not to increase chances of falling pregnant.

Although there isn't a magical pill to increase your chances, here are some common sense actions you can take.

From the above figures, we expect that about half of recipients who are attempting to conceive via natural insemination (NI, i.e., sexual intercourse) would get pregnant after 3-4 cycles. We would expect more than 90% of recipients to fall pregnant after 12 cycles of trying to conceive with NI. In comparison, we expect that about half of women would get pregnant after 6-7 cycles with chilled, shipped semen. Therefore, when a recipient tries to conceive via shipping, she should plan to try for 6-7 cycles on average. If she plans on 6-7 cycles, she is less likely to become discouraged and quit when the first attempt doesn't succeed. Unfortunately, many women set their hearts on a first cycle success, and become discouraged and give up when that doesn't happen. Mentally prepare yourself with realistic expectations.

Don't miss any cycles! The biggest reason people fail is not from infertility but from giving up. Prepare yourself mentally. For many people, skipping a cycle is their way to give up without admitting they're giving up. First they skip one cycle, and then another. Then they never go back. Don't give up.

According to the Center for Disease Control's 2012 Assisted Reproductive Technology Report, by age 37 the success rate falls by about 25% versus what it was at 34; by 40, it falls by about 30% versus what it was at 37; by 42 it is only half what it was at 40, and it halves again by 44.

Time is not on your side if you're a recipient: you should start trying as soon as possible once you decide that this is what you want to do, and especially if you are over age 34, don't miss any cycles.

If you are overweight, it may take you longer also, but it is advisable to start trying to conceive first, possibly while engaging in moderate weight loss, rather than wait until you lose weight, especially if you are in your mid 30's or older. Even though it is better for your health and your future child's health to lose that weight, be realistic: if you have tried to lose weight unsuccessfully many times already, it may take you a long time to lose the weight, or you may never lose it, so if you wait, you may never become pregnant. A low impact diet and exercise regimen, such as walking for 30 minutes every day and not drinking anything but water, while trying to conceive is preferable to waiting or going on an extreme diet or fitness program.

If you smoke, try to stop, as tobacco and other substances can reduce fertility.

Don't self-medicate with gray market fertility drugs you bought on the internet. The side effects could interfere with your cycle, and poor quality drugs taken without a doctor's advice may not provide any therapeutic benefit.

Avoid shift work, or a lifestyle that keeps you up all night: get to bed every night at a reasonable time, and go to bed at the same time every night.

Place TTC in first place: don't let your anxieties, job, family members, friends, pets, hobbies, lifestyle, or other activities distract you from your focus. Believe it or not, your dedication to TTC can cause family and friends to become jealous and try to derail you, for example, by undermining your commitment to use a free donor through dire warnings of the dangers of meeting someone on the internet. I don't know of any recipients who have been injured by a donor. Donors are interested in helping you to achieve pregnancy and little else.

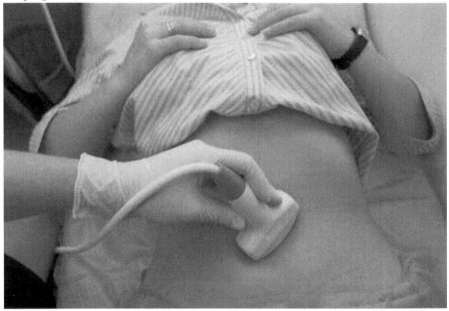

Chapter 3: Shipping chilled semen: an alternative to sperm banks

Sperm bank costs are prohibitive; services could easily cost $1,000.00 per insemination or more. They pass on the costs (along with a healthy profit) of expensive testing, preparation of semen, and freezing, which may or may not really be necessary, to the consumer. Since banks, due to regulatory requirements for expensive testing, have a monopoly, customers have no choice, allowing banks to maintain high rates. Private donors typically only pass on shipping expenses, and their shipping costs are much less, since they do not require heavy nitrogen tanks and the like that are necessary for banks.

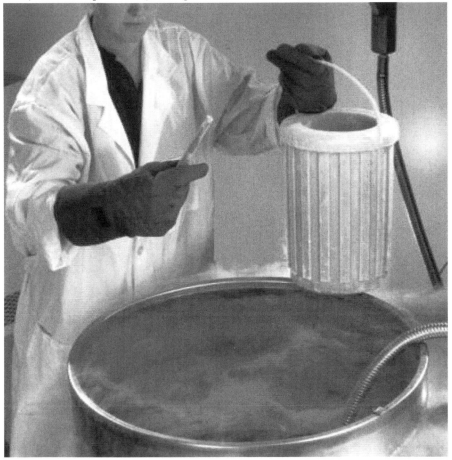

Women living in rural areas may have few or no local banks

Women living in rural areas may have few or no local banks, requiring travelling long distances. Air travel could cost a lot, as it is difficult to buy tickets until the last minute.

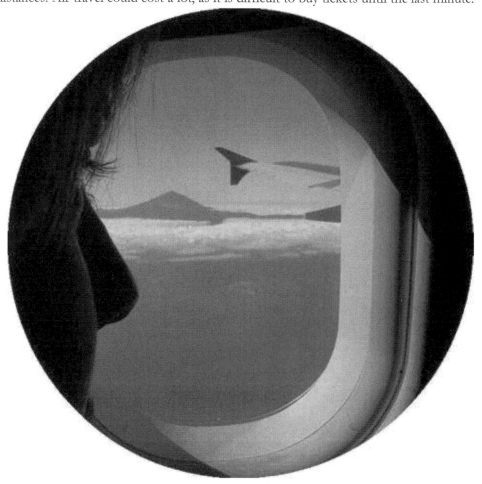

Recipients may have to undergo exams at sperm banks

New regulatory requirements may force recipients, who are not sick, to undergo testing, counseling, and exams that the millions of other mothers who do not use banks never have to undergo.

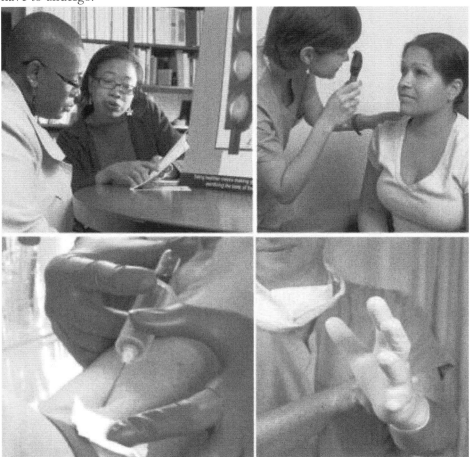

Some banks may even refuse to help single or gay women.
Some banks may have policies against helping single women, gay women, women with fertility issues, women with advanced maternal age, etc.

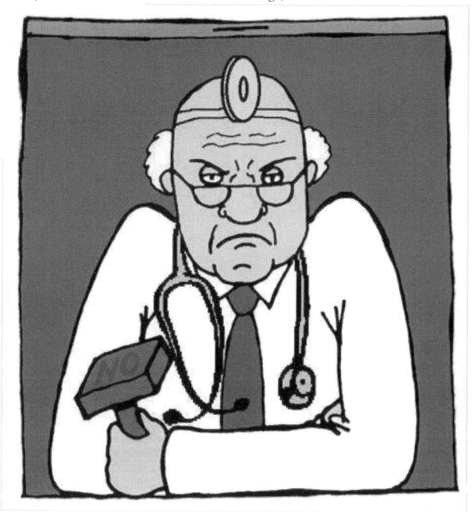

Why pay so much more for unnecessary poking and prodding?

Why pay so much more for unnecessary poking and prodding, invasion of privacy, and frozen "spermcicle" from a donor you will never meet when shipping chilled semen costs considerably less, is twice as effective as frozen, and is sent by a private donor you can talk to.

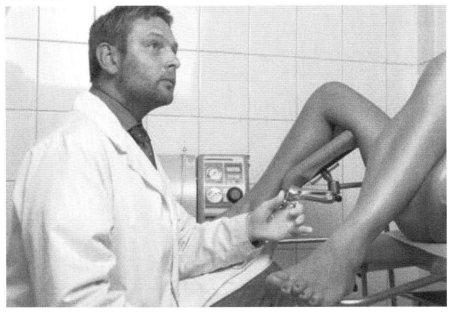

Banks offer airtight legal protection (at a price), but do you need it?

Banks also offer airtight legal protection to insure the recipient (and her partner where applicable) are the only legal parents. It may seem to recipients that private donors are risky in comparison, but other women who conceive outside of sperm banks have no guarantee that a baby daddy will not insinuate himself in to their life. With recent changes in the legislature on gay marriage, and acknowledgement of the spouse, even if the recipient's spouse is a woman, marriage is one way to guarantee that the partner will be the only other legal parent. A gay couple I helped in Virginia has already done this. Step-parent adoptions can also be done easily without recourse to a lawyer in many jurisdictions. A woman I helped in Connecticut who is remarrying is doing this. These methods are also airtight.

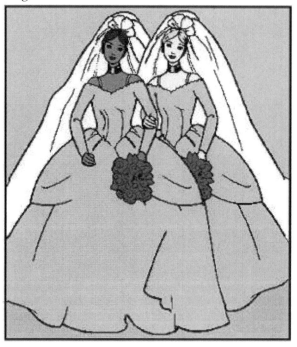

Does the legal protection offered by a bank justify the cost?

A recipient can also conceal her identity (methods explained in this book) to some degree if she is still worried. As is often said, "possession is nine tenths of the law," and the recipient will clearly have the child. Shipping donors are usually far away and have their own lives outside donation, if they are popular donors they may already have dozens of other children, they simply are not going to fight an uphill legal battle to get access to a faraway child they have no connection with. On the other hand, we see private sperm donations becoming more common, with courts developing precedents of how to deal with them, at the same time seeing the airtight promises of sperm banks being eroded by suits from donor children trying to find their donor fathers. The differences between legal options between banks and private arrangements are collapsing. I personally know hundreds of women who conceived with private donors with no legal problems. Donors generally do not want an active role in raising the child; otherwise they would not become donors. Legal protections offered by a bank are nice but when the actual situation is considered logically and in light of experience as a donor, I wonder if they are necessary enough to warrant the additional cost.

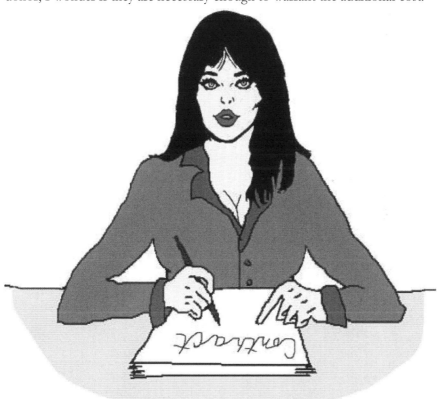

Private donors offer greater selection

Not all sperm freezes well. Banks reject significant percentages of applicants whose sperm does not freeze well. For them the donor's number one quality is sperm freezability, but this does not guarantee personality or good looks. Banks like tall donors who have a PhD, since those are easily quantified features that appeal to many women. Skin, hair and eye color are also easily described, but physical attractiveness and social intelligence are not quantifiable: he could easily be tall, smart, unattractive, and socially awkward. There are also few minority donors available at banks. However, if you want to use a private donor, you can select from amongst hundreds of private donors who advertise on the internet. You can email, see pictures, talk on the phone, even video chat on Skype, Oovoo, Facebook and the like, to decide for you if he is a good match for looks and personality. There is also a wider selection of minority donors available: I know a half dozen Asian, African American, and Latino donors on the sites I frequent. There are probably just as many ways to select a prospective donor for one's children as there are recipients: everyone will have their own criteria. However, since you are looking for someone to ship chilled semen, in addition to the traits you want for a potential donor in general, you would want one who has shipping successes and is familiar with the technical concepts that are discussed in this guide.

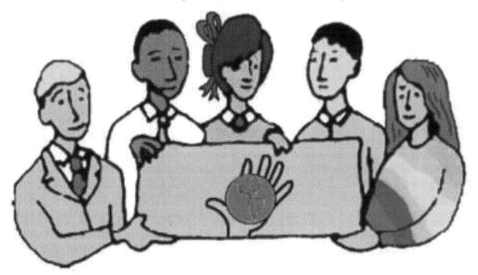

Chapter 4: How can I protect my privacy?

As a recipient, you may want to know a lot about your donor, but you may also want to control what he knows about you. Especially with shipping, he must have a street address and a phone number to send your semen by overnight express mail, so there are some limits on what you can do, but these things may make you feel better. "If you cannot trust your donor, you may want to choose someone else," is a good rule of thumb. However, although I have never known of any recipient who came to harm due to her donor knowing her name, address, and phone number, I know some women do become very nervous even if the donor is quite reliable. If it worries you, here are a few simple things you can do to make yourself feel more comfortable.

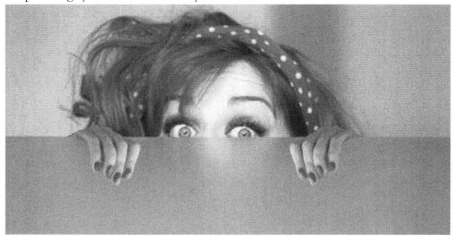

Will my donor know my home address?

For your donor to ship to you, you need to give him a phone number and a street address to ship to, but you can still conceal your home address. I have never known of any recipient who came to harm due to her donor knowing her home address, but if it worries you, it is nice to know you have a few options. You cannot overnight to a PO Box at the U.S. Post Office, so you cannot use a PO Box in place of your home address. You can, however, get a box at "The UPS Store" or other mailbox store (as I am in the USA, I am using the U.S. company UPS as an example; if you are not in the USA, or you are in the USA and want to use a different company, many of the principles I discuss are still going to apply, you would just have to check yourself with the company you use). Unlike a U.S. Post Office PO Box, boxes at these stores do count as street addresses. Just be sure to not call it a "PO Box" in your shipping address. But he might just Google my name, you say? Especially if you have a common legal name like (Brown, Smith, etc.) a Google search will not reveal much, if he does not have other information. You can use a business name, a middle name, a nickname, a maiden name, etc., in your shipping address if your legal name is likely to come up in a Google search. You may want to let the mailbox provider know you will receive mail under those names. Without a subpoena, UPS will not release your real address or name to anyone. You can also use a mailbox provider who is in a different zip code to lessen the chance a Google search will link your name to your home address. Just insure it is not so far away that you cannot get shipments in time.

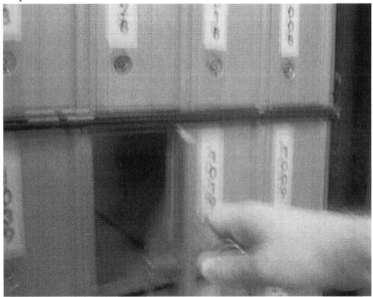

Do you want semen delivered here?

Even if you are not worried about your donor knowing where you live, getting a box at The UPS Store may be a good option if you: live in a low-rent area and do not want vagabonds rummaging through your semen shipment should it arrive while you are not home; you live in a rural area with uncertain delivery and do not want it to sit in the back of the ups truck in 100-dgree heat all day; you move frequently and do not want it sent to an old address by mistake; or you do not want the delivery person, who delivers to you and your neighbors and may know a lot about the community you live in, to know about your packages. Donors usually send non-descript packages, but still, one cannot be too careful.

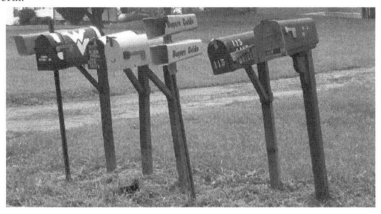

Always have UPS leave the package without signature

You should always have UPS leave the package at your door without signature, otherwise, some drivers who may not knock too hard on the door, might take your package back to the office thinking you are not home, in which case you are unlikely to get the package in time to inseminate that day and many sperm will die. Always authorize UPS to leave the package without a signature in order to avoid this issue. You can also leave instructions for UPS to leave the package in the shade, to leave in a particular place by your home, etc.

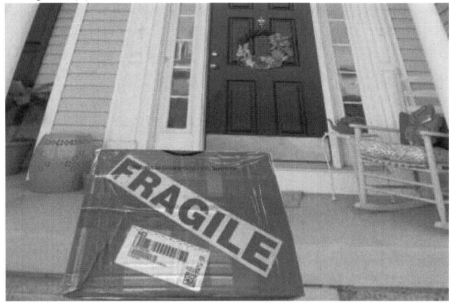

No UPS box, no problem

You can also ask your donor to ship to a local "The UPS Store" or UPS Service Center if you have one nearby, and have UPS hold it for you. Even if you do not have a box there, the store will be happy to do this for you. It is something to keep in mind if you are visiting friends or relatives during your fertile period and still want to inseminate. In theory the store clerk could ask for id when you pick up, so you may want your name to match, or at least have a non-suspicious reason (nick name, middle name, maiden name, etc.) why your ID and the name on the package are different. Why the name on the label does not match your id. However, in practice they often do not ask for id. If the package is being held at the ups store, and especially if the name on the label is not a complete match with your id, you would want to make sure you have given your donor a working phone number to put on the label.

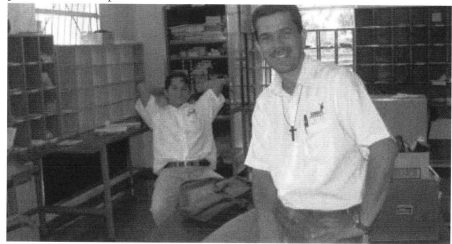

What about my Facebook identity?

Our Facebook group (facebook.com/groups/JoesDonorGroup) is "private" so that nonmembers cannot see messages posted there. However, if you join with your Facebook profile that family and friends use to communicate with you, then, when you make new friends on the donor group who are obviously identified in their profiles as sperm donors, they may get invites to connect with your friends from "real life" who may not realize you are using a donor, or vice versa. If you have 500+ friends it is possible no one will notice. Or, if you are gay and many of your friends are also using donors, it may not be a problem. Using a real Facebook profile makes donors very comfortable helping you since they know you are a real person. However, if for example you are married and your husband's infertility is not common knowledge, you may prefer the anonymity of a new account. If you make a Facebook profile only for donation, be sure to use an email address that you never used before: just make a new free Gmail or Yahoo account. This eliminates the risk a real life acquaintance you emailed in the past will get a recommendation from Facebook to friend your new donor friends.

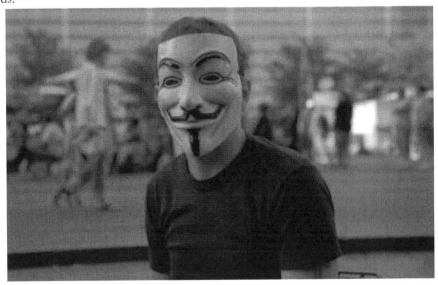

What about my phone number?

You must use a phone number for express deliveries. Although I have never known this to be a problem, if giving out your number worries you, there are simple things you can do. In some cases I have had to ship without knowing the recipient's phone number, so I put my own phone number on the label, but you may not want to do this when picking up at the ups store, especially if your id does not match. It is also more likely the ups store might call if they are holding your package, so recipients may want to have a working number that appears on the package. To easily get a working number that is not connected to you, you can get a pre-paid phone, such as a TracFone, with cash at Wal-Mart or many convenience stores. You never need give a name and it can cost as little as $20. Some people also get free disposable numbers on the internet (for example Google Voice) but to me seems like a TracFone would be more reliable, in case the express mail company or your donor really need to get in touch with you about your package when you are not on the internet.

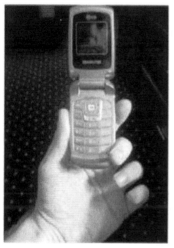 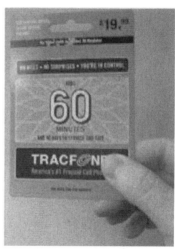

Chapter 5: How to time your insemination

Sperm is known to survive in the female reproductive track for up to five days. This information is an outside limit, used in family planning to prevent unwanted pregnancies by avoiding intercourse in the timeframe sperm could be expected to survive into a woman's fertile times. It is also used in forensic medicine, to determine when a sex crime may have taken place. However, for our purposes, we are interested in the timeframe that sperm is able to impregnate the egg, which is a much shorter time period, 24 to 48 hours at the most. When you ship, the sperm has usually been in the box for 12-18 hours of its useful life already and timing is even more essential.

Once a donor is selected, the first thing the recipient should do is determine when her last cycle day 1 (cd1) was, and tell her donor, so they can predict when to start doing OPK (ovulation prediction kit) testing and when he will need to be ready to ship.

Cd1 is the day AF starts (first day of period, first day of bleeding). In TTC (trying to conceive) parlance, we often refer to the period as "Aunt Flow" (AF). The average cycle is 28 days (cd1-cd28), but there is variance between women, even between cycles in the same women. Cycles may lengthen with age, some women with polycystic ovary syndrome (PCOS) may have significantly longer cycles, and some women with luteal phase defect may have shorter cycles. It is good for a recipient to share factors that affect your timing with her donor. It is a good idea to plan out estimated cycle events as soon as AF starts and to send any funds the donor needs so he can purchase supplies in time.

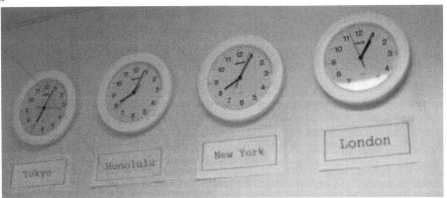

What is an OPK? What is the LH surge?

The ovulation prediction kit (OPK) is a test that detects HCG (human chorionic gonadotropin) that is released during the woman's luteinizing hormone (LH) surge. The LH surge causes ovulation to take place, and ovulation usually follows 12-36 hours after the surge.

A positive on the OPK does not actually indicate ovulation; it only indicates that the LH surge, which triggers ovulation, has occurred. Ovulation usually happens the day after the positive OPK. You will want to ship overnight on the day of the positive OPK, to arrive the next day. I have had successes two days after the positive OPK, perhaps that was a case of ovulation happening 36 hours later, and the egg living for 24 hours after that, and pregnancy could well result if ovulation was only 12 hours after the positive when shipping the day before the positive, as people sometimes do when expecting a positive on a weekend, but I believe it is best to ship the day of the positive OPK.

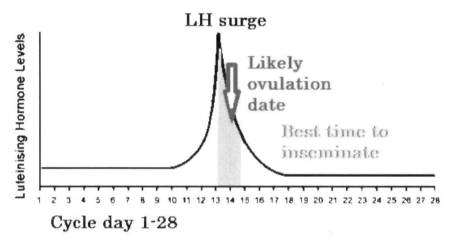

What should I do if I get two positives on the OPK in the same cycle?

Every now and then, a woman will tell me she got a positive OPK, I ship, and then a few days later, she reports a second positive. I believe there are several reasons this happens.

1. The first "positive" was not really a positive. She just jumped the gun. Be sure to read the test instructions carefully, as with some tests, the test line must be darker than the control line, whereas on others it need only be as dark as. It may be necessary to experiment with different brands, since a brand that consistently gives you multiple positives may be too sensitive for you.

2. The first positive was in fact correctly detecting an LH surge. However, the LH surge was insufficient to trigger ovulation, and a few days later a second surge occurred that actually triggered ovulation.

3. The second positive was the ovulation of a second egg. If you get mittelschmerz (ovulation pains) that are typically on one side of the body, and you felt it on the left the first time and on the right the second time, or vice versa, it is possible you are ovulating a second time.

In any of these three cases, you would want to ship again with the second OPK.

4. You are taking a hormone-based drug or supplement that is causing a false positive. In this case, stop taking the product or see your doctor for advice on how to time insemination.

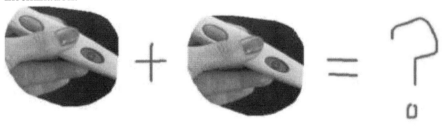

Timing of typical cycle events

In my experience women get a positive ovulation prediction kit (OPK) result anywhere between cd9-cd15. The hCG of the LH surge that is detected by the test may only last a few hours, and could easily pass unobserved in the 23 hours between tests if a recipient only tests once a day. So, I recommend one take the OPK twice a day starting on cd9. On average, women get a positive on cd13 most often, sometimes cd12, and less frequently on cd9-cd11, cd14-15.

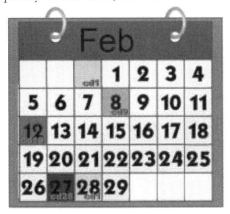
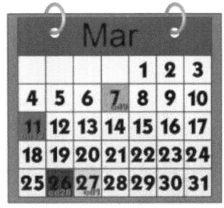
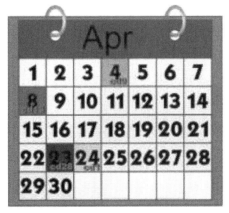

Use paper calendar not computer program

Cycle events tend to fall on the same day of the week, week after week, since the average cycle length, 28, is divisible by seven, it will line up very well with your calendar. We need to stop thinking of cycles as being synonymous to months, since they are not 28-days long or divisible by seven, and think in terms of weeks.

I advise against using computer or smart phone aps. Get a paper calendar and write things down: work, school, business hours, etc. Are organized weekly, and so is the menstrual cycle, seeing it on a calendar in that format is very intuitive. You will be planning around work schedules, school schedules, and business hours for shipping companies and mail deliveries. Besides, TTC is at heart an analog event.

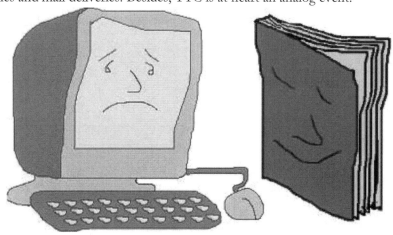

Cd1 never same day two months in a row

When a recipient says, "I track my cycles, cd1 comes every month on the 5th", I know she is not really tracking it and does not know what her cycle looks like on a calendar. Unless the month is 28 days long (only three out of every 48 months is 28 days long, that being February except leap year), it is unlikely cd1 would arrive on the same day of the month two months in a row, since 45 out of 48 months are longer than 28 days, the next cd1's day of the month would be 2-3 days sooner in the month than the preceding one. If it was the 5th this month, I would expect it to be the 2nd or the 3rd of the following month. What is more important than the day of the month is if she is actually tracking it, and if it is going to fall on a weekend every month and cause conflicts with express delivery, or always conflict with someone's work or school.

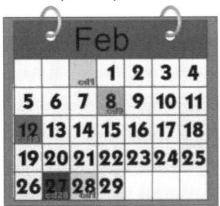
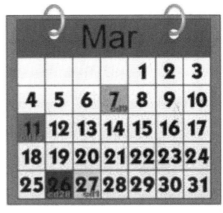
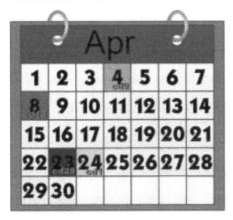

Practical example

In this example, a recipient's cd1 (first day period bleeding) falls on Jan 31. She estimates future cd1's (Feb 28, & Mar 27), cd9's (start OPK testing: Feb 8 & Mar 7), cd13's (likely positive OPK/LH surge and best insem days: Feb 12 & Mar 11), and cd28's (hpt test dates: Feb 27 & Mar 26). She will revise march estimates based on when her next AF starts, but she can estimate march dates from Jan 31 for planning purposes.

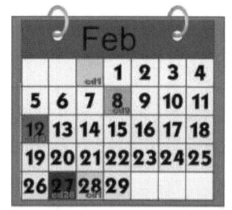
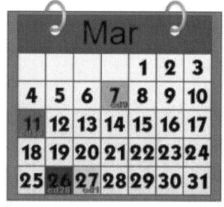
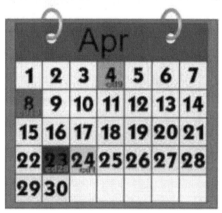

Chapter 6: The OPK (ovulation prediction kit)

Some OPK tests use a chemically treated strip that is dipped in urine that has been collected in a cup. With some other OPK tests, urine is collected in a cup and then dropped into the tester using a sterile pipette. Then there are some OPK tests that can be inserted in to the urine stream directly. This type can usually also be dipped in a cup of urine.

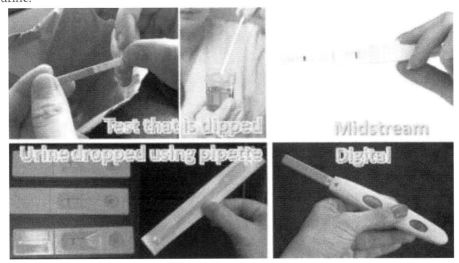

Reading test results on the OPK

OPK positive test results almost always require the test (t) line to be equally dark as the control (c) line, and sometimes it must be darker. Carefully read instructions! If the control line does not show, the test is invalid. Some people prefer a digital test, but the non-digital shows fade-ins (test line present but not darker than control) that can indicate that ovulation is on the way. Try several brands to see which works best for you.

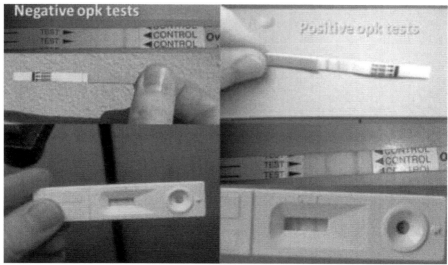

The Clearblue Advanced Digital Ovulation Test

According to Clearblue's website, "The Clearblue Advanced Digital Ovulation Test is a breakthrough: not only does it detect the rise in LH, it also monitors the level of another key fertility hormone, estrogen, which increases in the days before the LH surge. Because your partner's sperm can survive in your body for up to 5 days, you can actually become pregnant by having intercourse during the days leading up to ovulation. By tracking these 2 key hormones, this test is able to typically identify 4 fertile days leading up to, and including the day of ovulation, twice as many as any other ovulation tests." (The below screenshot from a promotional video on the website illustrates the theory).

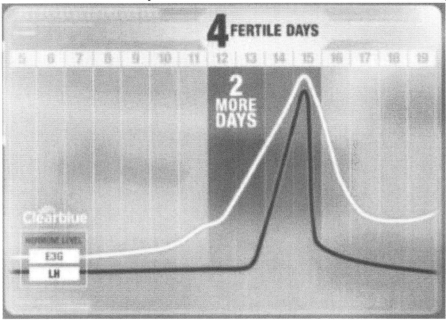

This sounds good in theory, except that the woman is not actually fertile for four days. The egg lasts about 24 hours. She is fertile for maybe one day. The theory proposed by Clearblue is that since some sperm may hypothetically survive 4-5 days, an insemination 4-5 days prior to ovulation will hypothetically result in the survival of sperm until the one day that the woman is actually fertile. The theory that sperm live 4-5 days is based on forensic medicine, in which the presence of live sperm is used as an indicator that ejaculation, and any crime related to the ejaculation, occurred within the preceding 4-5 days. That is not to say that those sperm still alive in the vagina are still able to fertilize an egg. For one thing, if the sperm is still in the vagina, it is probably defective, since it never passed through the cervix and never made it to the egg. In my experience, insemination must be done the day of the positive ovulation test or the day after the positive ovulation test. This test might be useful in giving you advanced warning (the way that fade-ins on the conventional ovulation tests give you advanced warning), but, especially for shipping, since the sperm is shipped overnight, and expends half its useful life in transit, it isn't going to live as long as fresh sperm would in the woman's reproductive tract, so it isn't realistic to expect a pregnancy to result from inseminations done during the first two days of the so-called "4 fertile days." Here is a picture of a "peak fertility" result on the Clearblue Advanced Digital Ovulation Test from a successful insemination.

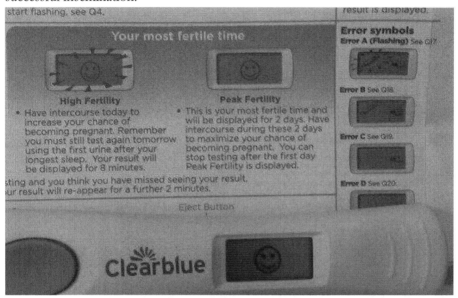

She also did a conventional ovulation test that same day and got a positive:

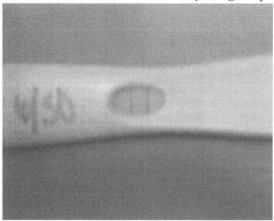

The recipient was far away, it took 24 hours for me to get to her, but she fell pregnant after an insemination done on the second "peak fertility" day, corresponding to the day after the positive ovulation test on a conventional test. For a fertile couple that lives together, inseminating four days in a row isn't going to hurt. However, for a recipient who has to arrange insemination with a donor, and may not have four days to play with, she has to focus on the "peak fertility" days, and the so-called "high fertility" days (I think "high fertility" is misleading: if anything these are "low fertility" days) are probably only useful as an early warning that the actual fertile days is 2-3 days away.

Chapter 7: Using basal temperatures to predict ovulation

Some 20 years ago when I first started to try to conceive (TTC), basal temperatures, along with cervical mucus and change in cervical position, were the standard tools for predicting ovulation. Basal temperatures were instrumental in conceiving one of my children. This method requires much discipline, you must take a basal temperature each morning at the same time before getting out of bed to urinate and go to bed and wake up at about the same time every day. It is not always suitable to younger individuals' hectic lifestyles today. The book "Taking Charge of Your Fertility" explains basal temps in detail.

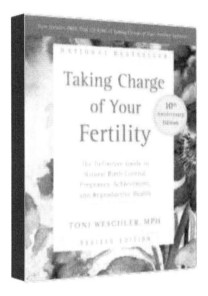

You will probably need to chart a few cycles in order to get good results. Remember, the basal thermometer measures in tenths of degrees (I have seen some women do not realize that). The OPK is so much more convenient and readily available at the dollar store for $1, or online for less. I would advise doing basal temperatures as an ancillary method to help when OPK results are difficult to interpret.

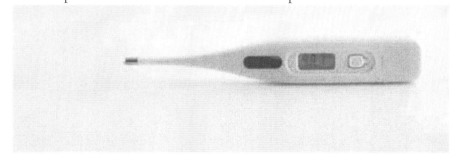

You can see in this example there is a slight rise on cd14, a noticeable dip on cd15, then a steep rise. That pattern is indicative of ovulation. The slight rise on cd14 is probably due to the LH surge, with the steep rise that follows it due to ovulation. Temperatures remain high past cd28, and then climb to a new plateau about cd33. That pattern is most surely pregnancy. A precipitous drop about cd28 would be indicative of the start of a new cycle.

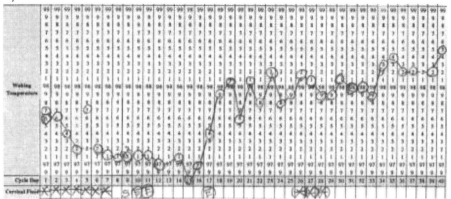

Chapter 8: Predict ovulation from change in the cervix

Some 20 years ago when I first started TTC, change in cervical mucus and change in the cervix, along with basal temperatures, were standard tools for predicting ovulation. However cervical changes were lesser partners to basal temps. You must check about the same time each day, with your body in about the same position, to get the best results, and it requires a few cycles to get accustomed to it.

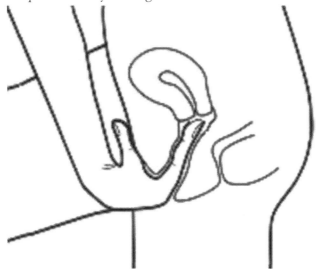

Mucus especially can also be affected by other factors such as hydration or cough medicine, etc. I have not found this method to be reliable with many women I help. There is a tendency to predict ovulation several days earlier than it shows on the OPK. In my opinion the OPK is the best option for shipping. The book "Taking Charge of Your Fertility" explains the use of cervical changes in detail.

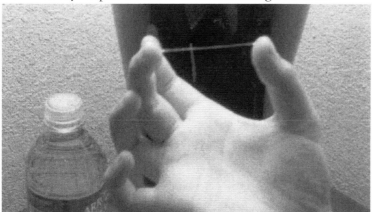

Some women view the cervix through a speculum to see if it is open or closed. The key is to view the changes in the cervix throughout the cycle, to see how it changes as key cycle dates approach. The book "Taking Charge of Your Fertility" explains in detail.

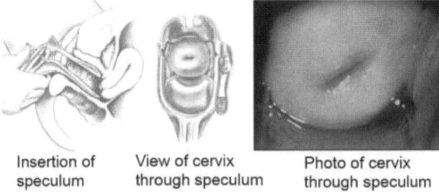

Insertion of speculum   View of cervix through speculum   Photo of cervix through speculum

The "Beautiful Cervix Project" (www.beautifulcervix.com) has a great collection of free images of the cervix to help you decipher your results. Basically, you should be examining the cervix looking for changes that precede the LH surge, which you verify on the ovulation test, so that you can better predict when ovulation will occur and plan for holidays, weekends, and the like with your donor.

Chapter 9: Predicting ovulation with mittelschmerz and other ways

Some women experience mittelschmerz, a medical term for ovulation pain that is derived from the German word for "middle pain". Typically it will occur on only one side. I have known several women to rely on this to time insemination successfully. Through careful tracking of cycles, especially older women may become aware of ovulation-related pains or twinges that can serve as reliable ovulation symptoms.

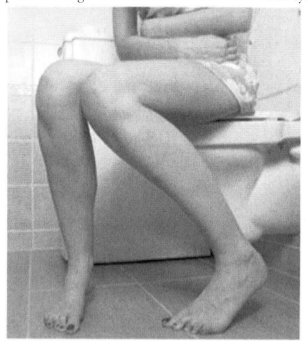

Other ways to predict ovulation

There are ovulation monitors, such as the OvaCue, they cost more than the OPK, but I do not see them working better than the OPK. Keep in mind that in addition to the monitor, you must often buy refill cartridges for it. They are most useful for women who do not respond well to the OPK. Since for TTC we are interested in the LH surge more than ovulation, the OPK (actually an LH surge predictor) seems better suited. It can be confusing to work with an ovulation monitor after using the OPK. The OvaCue is well known and available online. You can also find ovulation microscopes for looking at ferning, such as Fertile Focus, online.

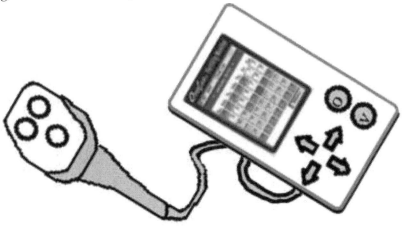

Chapter 10: Summary of key cycle dates

On cd1, send donor funds so he can order supplies.

On cd9, begin testing with the OPK, twice daily, 10am and in the pm. Make sure the pm testing is before the last UPS or FedEx truck leaves, usually around 4-5pm.

On day of the positive OPK, usually about cd12-13, inform your donor immediately so he can prepare the sample. Test at 10am and again in the pm, leaving time for him to get to the express mail company before their last truck leaves, usually around 4-5pm.

At 14 days after the positive OPK, usually about cd28, do the HPT (home pregnancy test). Be sure to inform your donor of results ASAP so he can plan for next cycle, to help you again if negative, or to help someone new if your test is positive. You can test as early as 10dpo, but may get false negatives.

Note: The day your period ends (the day you stop menstrual bleeding) is NOT important to TTC. It often happens about cd3-7, too early to interfere with TTC. There is no need to track this date or to discuss with your donor, there are already many dates to keep track of, and it just adds confusion.

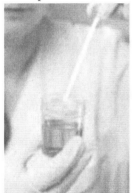
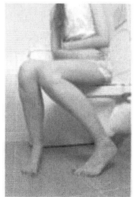
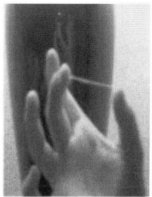

Chapter 11: TYB, shipping kits, and collecting and shipping semen

TYB (test yolk buffer) is a semen extender that is marketed by Irvine Scientific. The semen extender is the essential ingredient for shipping. It nourishes the semen, buffers it against cold shock, and contains antibiotics that control the bacteria that naturally occur in the semen. These bacteria are probably harmless to humans, but if semen sits around too long, the bacteria can proliferate, and their toxic byproducts kill or degrade semen, so many extenders include an antibiotic. You should not use TYB if you are allergic to eggs, antibiotics, and the like. In addition to the semen extender, a typical shipping kit may also include sterile, individually wrapped syringes, individually wrapped sterile pipettes, insulated foil envelopes, sterile specimen cups, nitrile gloves, cold packs, transport vials, and Softcups, often in an insulating Styrofoam box with outer cardboard carton. There are variations between different kits, but, aside from the semen extender, it isn't especially difficult to obtain the other contents of the kit.

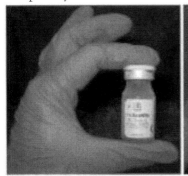 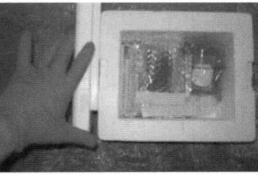

Cold packs

Be sure to freeze the cold packs beforehand. Freeze them flat so they fit better in the box. Bags will eventually break (especially the Uline cold packs, which are meant for a single use), so don't recycle, spend a little more to use a new bag and avoid a leaky package, which could be catastrophic in today's security-conscious environment, since the package might be held, opened for inspection, and UPS or FedEx might try very hard to get in touch with all parties concerned to find out what is in the package (if you did not announce to them it was "semen"). Understandably, for donors who wish to remain anonymous, this type of attention is less than desirable. The cold packs below were obtained from a U.S. company called Uline. Uline cold packs come in different sizes, depending on how you use them, smaller sizes are sometimes more convenient, although the larger ones seem to thaw slower.

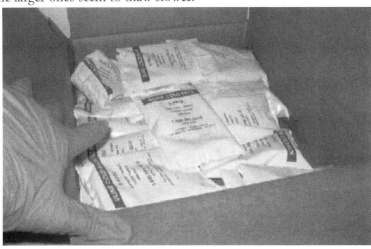

Other cold pack manufacturers

You can easily obtain cold packs at Target, Walmart, and similar stores. Your local supermarket and also hardware stores will often carry them as well. They may be described as "substitute ice" or other ways in addition to "cold packs". You will usually find them by the Styrofoam coolers in stores. Cost is typically under $2, or you may even get a set with individual prices that are even lower. (The Uline pack here is one of the smaller ones.)

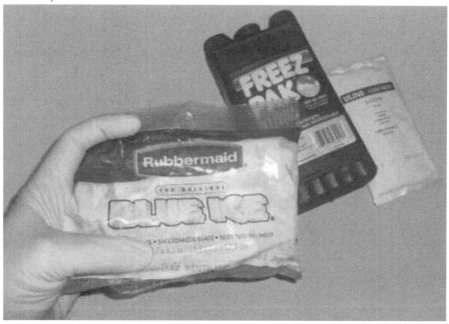

What do the recipients do with the parts of the kit after they inseminate?

The recipients in the USA never return the shipping kit. I wondered what they did with it. One woman said that her dog ate the kit. One said her husband uses the Styrofoam box to keep worms when he goes fishing. I saw on Facebook that another recipient used the cold pack to treat her child's injured hand. How funny that the cold pack would survive to be used on the hand of the child that was conceived using the kit! But they don't seem to return them. Donors may also not want to have the kit returned. Donors probably need to make a new kit for every shipment, so keep this in mind when calculating how much it costs to ship.

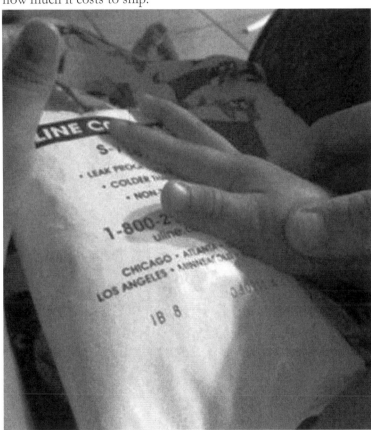

Specimen cup

Use a sterile, individually packaged specimen cup to collect the semen. If you use a non-sterile container, be sure that after washing it is well rinsed with hot water: soap residue may be more harmful to the semen than whatever was in the container before it was washed.

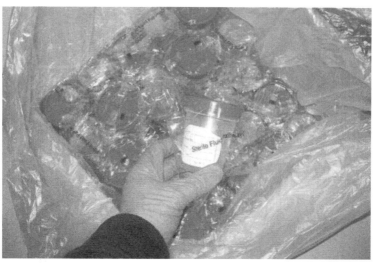

Sperm-Friendly Lubricant

If lubricant is necessary, use a non-spermicidal one, such as pre-seed.

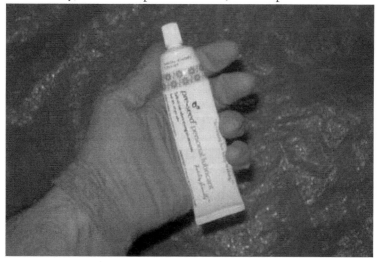

The sample, when collected, is coagulated

You must let it liquefy, usually takes 5-10 minutes, if it is coagulated it may not mix well with the semen extender. You can pass it through a pipette or 18-gauge syringe needle a few times to liquefy it if it is still too viscous to mix with the semen extender and you have no time to wait. Bubbles are normal.

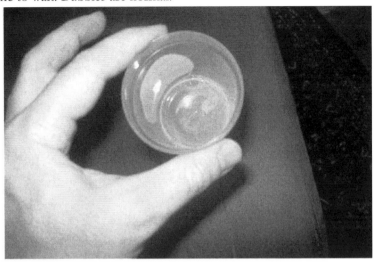

What Does Normal Volume Look Like?

Normal volume range for ejaculate is 2.5-5.0ml. The lowest graduation on this specimen cup is 20ml. As you can see, the ejaculate occupies about one fourth of the space below the 20ml graduation in the cup, or about 5ml. The syringe is about 5.5ml, the upper end of the normal range. This is when the donor collects it: when the recipient receives it, it will be twice as much, or about 10ml, since he will have added the extender in equal volume.

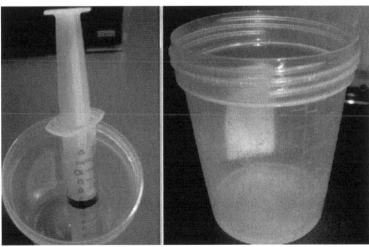

You may also collect with a Ziploc bag

If you do not have a sterile specimen cup, you may also use a new Ziploc bag that has been approved by the FDA for food use. It is not sterile, but, since it is approved for food use, the bag is made so that it won't leach harmful chemicals into food (or semen). Sometimes the thinner bags for making sandwiches are better, depending on how one goes about the collection. To get the semen out of the bag, wait for it to liquefy, and snip a corner off the bag and pour it from the hole, or use a syringe or pipette to aspirate the semen from the bag. The bag in the picture has perhaps a little over 5ml of semen. Bubbles are normal.

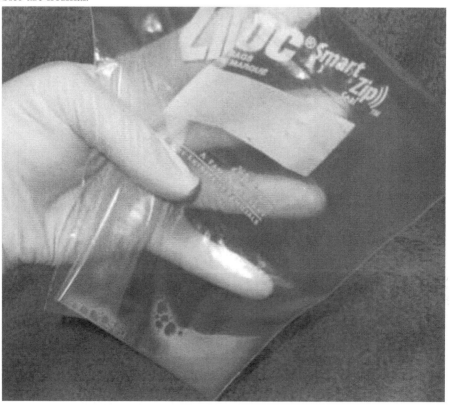

Chapter 12: The Semen Extender

The extender is the key element of the shipping kit. All other contents can be assembled fairly easily from numerous vendors, although especially for neophytes, it is much easier to have them all assembled together in a kit. The best known extender is Irvine Scientific's test yolk buffer (TYB), but Irvine will not sell directly to individuals, only to medical facilities. Rainbow Health Services sells complete kits that include Irvine's TYB. Cabrimed is selling its own extender that is for diagnostics use only and perhaps not approved for use in human insemination, although it apparently keeps the sperm alive. Baby Dust Delivery sells kits with extender or extra extender without the kit, but it seems to be their in-house formula and is not Irvine TYB.

I am not surprised if, in the future, more legal restrictions are placed on human semen extenders. Already the FDA considers Irvine's TYB to be a "medical device," which is why it is difficult to obtain. There doesn't really seem to be any medical reason for this restriction, other than attempts by the established medical industry to maintain its monopoly.

Semen needs to be buffered from pH and supported in a nutrient rich extender to survive for 24 hours outside the body. The normal semen volume range for a healthy man is about 2.5-5ml, and an equal portion of semen extender is added, so the extender comes in 5-ml vials, to accommodate the upper range of normal ejaculates. Caution: Extender may contain egg, dairy and antibiotics (usually gentamycin). If you are allergic to eggs, dairy, or antibiotics ask your doctor if it is safe for you. Be careful opening the bottle, as there is a metal ring you must pull off that can be sharp and cut your fingers.

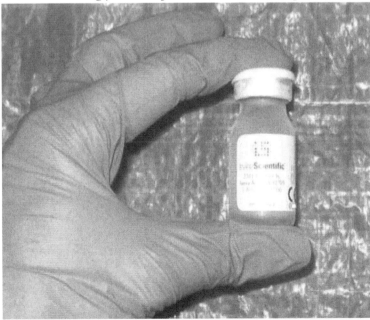

The manufacturer's directions for using Irvine TYB

1. Semen is collected following a two to three day abstinence period.

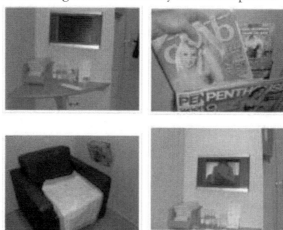

2. Sample is allowed to liquefy at 37°C for 30 minutes.

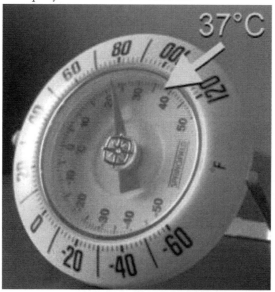

3. One vial of medium is thawed and brought to 37°C.

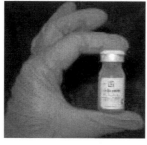

4. The liquefied sample is transferred to a sterile, 15 mL, conical centrifuge tube, the volume determined and medium added drop wise until a 1:1 sample: medium ratio is achieved.

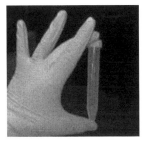

5. The sample-medium mixture is placed in a beaker or other suitable container of 37°C water.

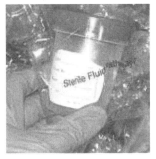

6. The container is refrigerated at 2°C to 5°C to allow a slow cooling of the mixture (0.5°C/minute).

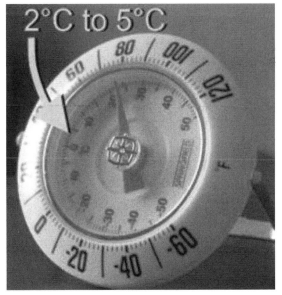

Open the TYB vial's metal lid using a knife

You can open the metal lid of the TYB vial by cutting it with a knife and pulling it off with pliers. Be careful not to cut your fingers. There is a rubber stopper under the metal lid that helps to prevent spillage when removing the metal lid.

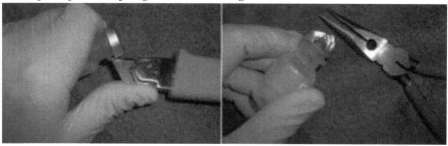

To mix semen and extender more thoroughly, use a pipette

Once the semen has liquefied, open up a sterile pipette. Add the semen and the extender in to a sterile specimen cup or similar container drop by drop: add one drop of semen, and then add one drop of extender. Gently swirl around to mix. To mix semen and extender even more thoroughly, use a pipette to aspirate the mixture of semen and extender in to the pipette then squirt it back into the container a few times. If you do not have a pipette, you can also pour the semen and extender in to a specimen cup or similar container, and then pour the mixture of semen and extender back and forth between the original cup and a second sterile specimen cup, or swirl the mixture around in the cup for a longer period.

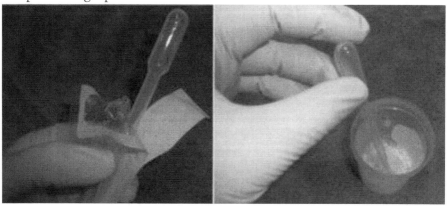

After thoroughly mixing the semen with the extender (TYB), transfer the mixture to one or more transport tubes.

Transport tubes can come in different sizes. Some women ask, "How many vials will you send?" This question is hard to answer, since vials come in various sizes. It is probably a question motivated by the sperm bank industry. They divide the donor's ejaculate in to several small portions, sometimes less than 1ml, so the recipient needs 2-3 vials in order to get pregnant. Free donors who ship chilled sperm send the entire ejaculate. Although ejaculate volume can vary between individuals, and the same individual may even produce different volumes at different times, the ejaculate will be of sufficient amount. So, this question isn't important.

Compare a 15-ml transport tube (left)to three 5-ml transport tubes (right): the number of vials isn't indicative of the actual amount of the sample.

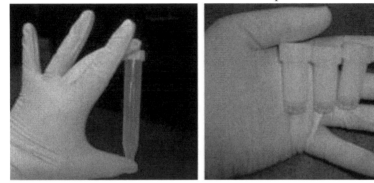

Water kills semen. Soap residue also kills semen.

If you must reuse containers, rinse thoroughly with hot water and dry very well. Water kills semen. Soap residue also kills semen. Rinsing with very hot water is probably good enough, without soap. Ideally don't reuse containers: always use a new, sterile implement. For syringes, pipettes, and catheters and the like, you may also rinse them out with physiological saline solution, as it will not harm the sperm the way that tap water would.

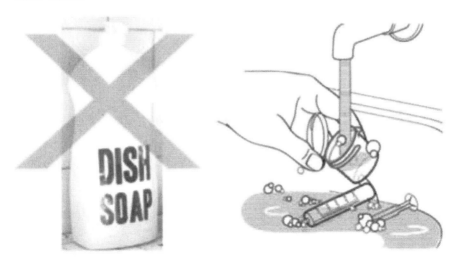

Chapter 13: Alternative to TYB: An extender made from powder

Liquid TYB must be sent to the donor frozen unless he plans to use it right away. After it thaws, it must be kept refrigerated and it must be used within two weeks. This is because the TYB is a rich nutrient, and it will spoil if it is not kept refrigerated. Even if TYB is kept refrigerated, eventually it will grow mold. This means that it is expensive to ship TYB to a donor, since it must be shipped by express mail and kept cold during shipping, and it is difficult to ship liquid TYB overseas due to the time required to ship overseas. Only small amounts can be shipped each time, since it will thaw, and the donor cannot usually use a large amount in two weeks. The powder, on the other hand, does not need to be refrigerated until it is mixed with the mixing solution (after it is mixed, it acts just like TYB, and must be kept refrigerated and used within two weeks, or frozen right after it is mixed). Therefore, the powder can be shipped less expensively and in greater volumes. It is also possible to ship it, for example, from the USA to the UK, Europe, Australia, or pretty much anywhere in the world. It is shipped to donors in nondescript packages, labeled as "protein powder" and "mixing solution." It is also possible to purchase a shipping kit (i.e. insulated Styrofoam box and other items necessary to ship) but, especially for international customers, the extender is the key ingredient, all other parts of the kit can be manufactured or obtained fairly easily.

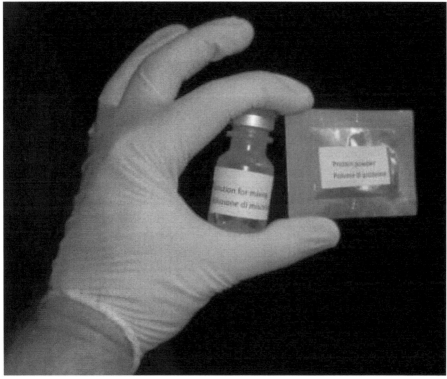

Prepare the powder extender

Open the mixing solution container. Sometimes it comes in a plastic vial with a screw top that is easy to open. Sometimes it comes in a vial with a metal lid. You can open the metal lid by cutting it with a knife and pulling it off with pliers. Be careful not to cut your fingers. There is a rubber stopper under the metal lid that helps to prevent spillage when removing the metal lid.

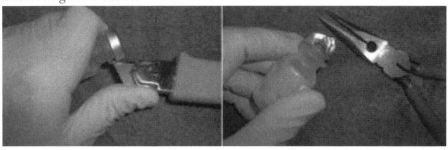

Prepare the powder extender

First pour the mixing solution into a sterile specimen cup or similar container.

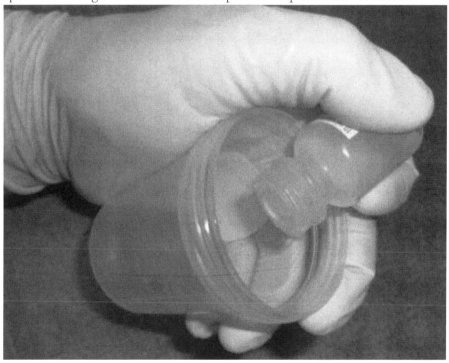

Cut open the small foil envelope containing the powder

(Sometimes the powder may come in a 5ml plastic vial with a screw top, in which case this step is not necessary).

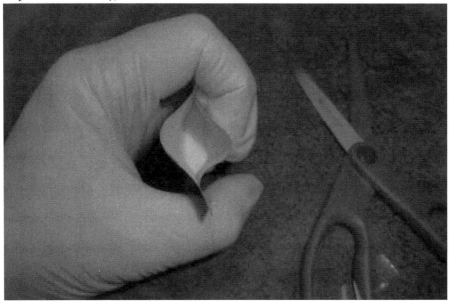

Dump the powder extender in to the container with the mixing solution.
Tap the bottom of the powder envelope (or other container) to make sure that all of the powder falls in to the mixing solution. Lightly tap the container to shake any powder from the walls of the specimen cup (or other container). Swirl the container to dissolve the powder. It dissolves easily. Many times the powder and solution come in a 10ml portion. You can divide the powder and solution in two before mixing, in which case the powder that is not mixed yet lasts longer. It is easier to divide the mixed solution than to divide the dry powder. If you expect to ship two ejaculates you can mix the entire 10ml and divide the mixed solution. After the powder tyb has been mixed, treat it the same as you would treat normal tyb. After it is mixed, you can store in the refrigerator for 2 weeks, or you can freeze it and it should keep for 1 year when frozen. This is what it looks like before dissolving. The prepared extender is a uniform translucent white after the powder is dissolved in the mixing solution.
(See this YouTube video on preparing the powder-based extender: http://youtu.be/9sduspWomrA)

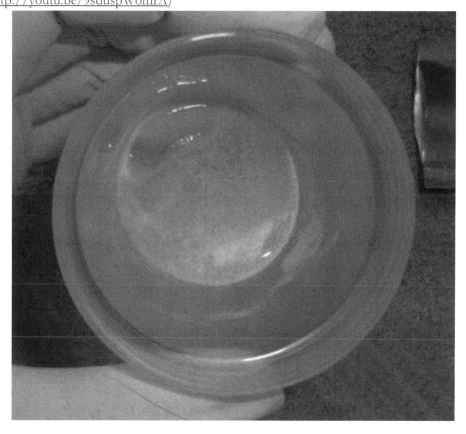

You can also pour the powder directly in to the mixing solution bottle

You can also prepare the powder extender by (carefully) pouring the powder directly in to the mixing solution bottle. Put the rubber stopper back on.

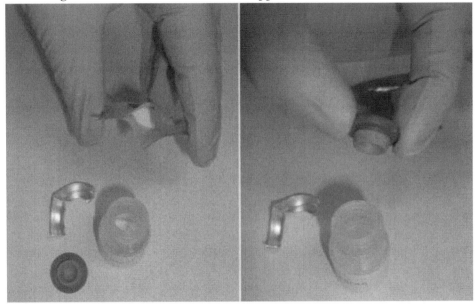

Shake the bottle in order to completely dissolve the powder in the mixing solution

Note that the bottle is 10ml, and if you have only 5ml of extender in the bottle (i.e. you kept back 5ml to use later), you can add the semen directly to the bottle, replace the stopper and metal lid, firmly tape it all shut again, and use for shipping the extended semen to the recipient.

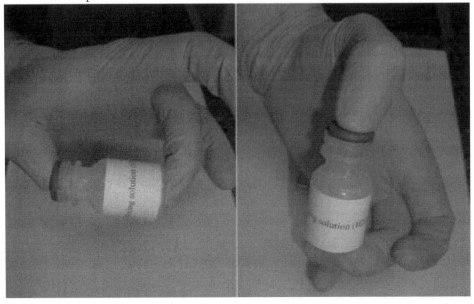

To mix semen and extender more thoroughly, use a pipette

Once the powder is dissolved in the mixing solution to form the extender, it behaves more or less like Irvine's TYB extender discussed above. Once the semen has liquefied, open up a sterile pipette. Add the semen and the extender in to a sterile specimen cup or similar container drop by drop: add one drop of semen, and then add one drop of extender. Gently swirl around to mix. To mix semen and extender even more thoroughly, use a pipette to aspirate the mixture of semen and extender in to the pipette then squirt it back into the container a few times. If you do not have a pipette, you can also pour the semen and extender in to a specimen cup or similar container, and then pour the mixture of semen and extender back and forth between the original cup and a second sterile specimen cup (or similar container), or swirl the mixture around in a single container for a longer period if you don't have a second container. After thoroughly mixing the semen with the extender transfer the mixture to one or more transport tubes. Ideally don't reuse containers, always use a new, sterile implement. If you must reuse containers, rinse thoroughly with hot water and allow to air dry. Dry very well, because tap water kills semen. Avoid soap, or rinse well, because soap residue also kills semen. You may also rinse items with physiological saline solution, as it will not harm the sperm the way that tap water would.

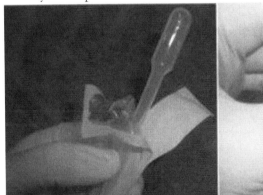 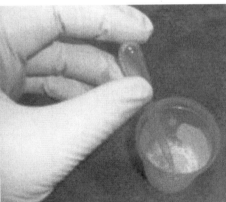

Sometimes the extender comes in a 10ml amount, with a bottle with 10ml of mixing solution and an envelope with enough powder for 10ml of extender.

You mix the mixing solution at a ratio of about 1:1 with semen. It is most convenient to prepare two portions of 5ml, which is enough for two ejaculates of 5ml each. An ejaculate is normally 2.5-5.0 ml. 10ml of the extender is enough for two shipments of 5ml each. If you mix 5.0ml of solution with an ejaculate of 2.5 ml, or a slightly larger than normal ejaculate of 5.5ml, that is acceptable. If the ejaculate for a particular donor is always about 3ml, I suppose you can separate the 10ml in to three portions of about 3ml each, but I would rather prepare two portions of 5ml to be certain to have enough for each ejaculate. You can divide 10ml of the extender in to smaller units before you mix the powder and mixing solution, or you can divide it in to smaller units after you mix the powder and mixing solution.

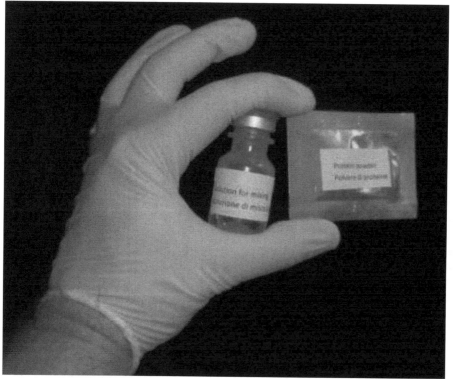

To divide extender powder in to 5ml portions before you mix the powder and mixing solution:

Pour the powder out on a smooth, dry, clean surface, such as a mirror for example. Divide the powder in to 5ml portions (if you have enough powder for 10ml of extender, then you would divide in to two evenly). You can use a thin, hard plastic card to divide the powder in to two lines of equal size. Typically a credit card is a little too thick; find a card that is thinner than that, such as this "Oyster" metro card from the UK.

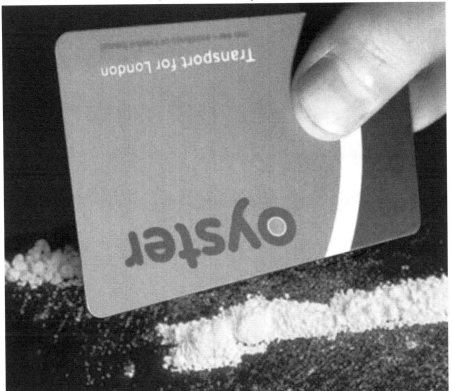

Keep the unused half of the powder in a small, sealed container in a cool, dry place

It does not need to be refrigerated. For example, keep the left over powder in an empty 5ml transport vial. Divide the mixing solution in half. A syringe can be used to measure out 5ml, or you can eyeball to see when the container is half-empty. Keep the unused half of the mixing solution in a small, sealed container in a cool, dry place. It does not need to be refrigerated. For example, pour half in to an empty 5ml transport vial.

Mix the 5ml of powder and 5ml of mixing solution to prepare 5ml of extender for immediate use.

You can keep the unused powder and unused mixing solution for 1 year in a cool, dry place. (Refrigeration is not necessary if it is still in powder form).

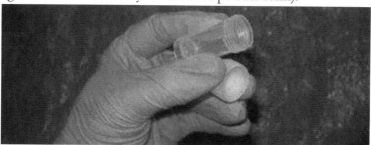

To divide after you mix the powder and mixing solution:

Mix the 10ml of mixing solution and the 10ml of powder normally. After they are mixed, pour 5 ml in to an empty 5ml transport vial. Since it is mixed, you should keep it refrigerated and use within 2 weeks. Or, you can freeze it immediately. Freezing may allow you to keep it for 1 year, but if you want to keep for one year, I recommend keeping it in an unmixed format, i.e., a powder and a mixing solution. You can thaw it by leaving it in the refrigerator for a few hours. After it thaws, you should keep it refrigerated and use within 2 weeks. It is a high nutrient solution. If you do not refrigerate it, it will spoil. If you refrigerate it longer than 2 weeks, it may also spoil. For example, mold may grow on it.

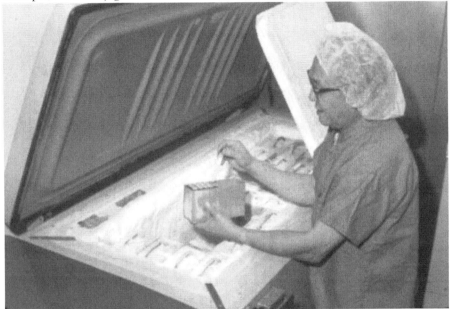

Chapter 14: Other contents of the kit: the transport vials

Since the sample size is about 2.5-5ml, and you add extender in equal amounts, you need at least two sterile 5-ml transport vials to accommodate total volumes in a range whose typical upper end is about 10.0ml. Vials come in many shapes. These 5-ml vials (right) have a screw cap to prevent spilling and a flat bottom that is stable for filling. The 15-ml vial (left), designed for use in a centrifuge, has an unstable, tapered bottom and must be held in hand or placed in a stand to keep it stable while filling it.
(YouTube video of the 15ml transport tube: http://youtu.be/9sduspWomrA)

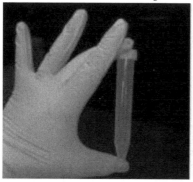
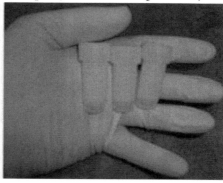

Two 5-ml vials may not be enough

In some cases, the ejaculate approaches or exceeds 5.0ml. The extender may also be slightly over 5.0ml in volume. Bubbles may form when filling the vial with the extended semen, causing it to occupy more space than it normally would and overflow out of the vial. In these cases, don't overfill the vial, simply use a third 5-ml vial.

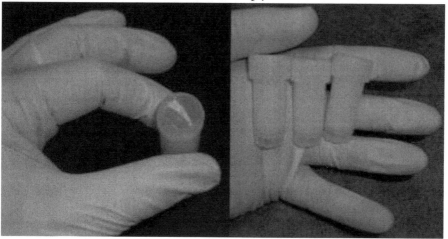

Sterile pipettes

Immediately after ejaculation semen is coagulated. Wait five to 10 minutes for the semen to liquefy. Then use a sterile, graduated pipette to transfer sample and equal amounts of TYB to the transport vials. Mix well so that all of the semen is properly buffered by the extender. To improve mixing, alternate dropping one drop of extender then one drop of semen using two pipettes. Further mix by gently rotating the vials (after firmly screwing on the caps) end over end for a few minutes. The pipette has a small mouth and the vacuum that is created can exert a surprising amount of force, so avoid creating a vacuum over sensitive skin.

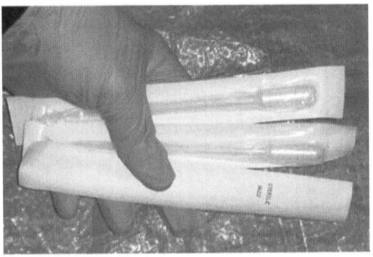

Insulated foil envelopes

Place the vials in an insulated foil envelope so they are not in direct contact with the cold packs.

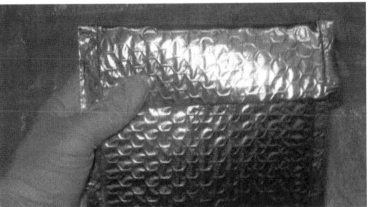

You can cut the insulated envelope in half if it is too large

Cutting the envelope in half also reduces expenses be economizing on the number if insulated envelopes that are used.

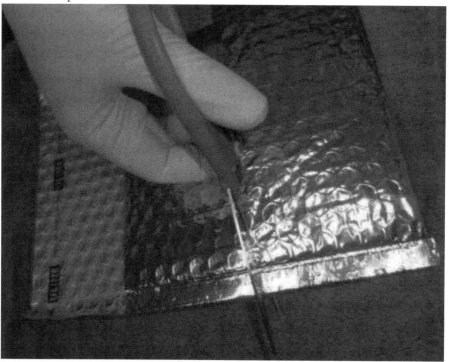

Place the vials of extended semen in the insulated envelope

If you cannot obtain an insulated envelope, you may also wrap the vials in paper towel and place in a Ziploc bag.

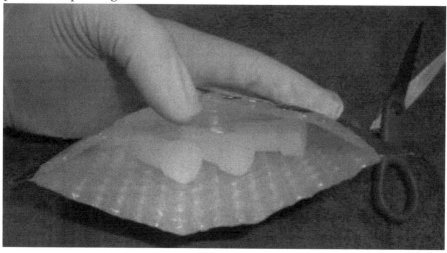

Close the envelope and tape it up with duct tape

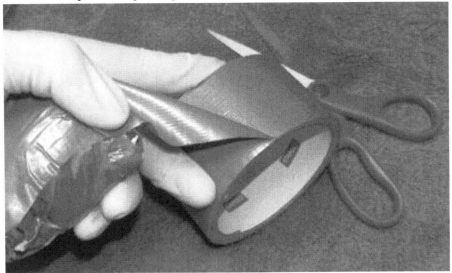

Individually wrapped sterile 10ml syringe

If an individually wrapped, sterile syringe is in the cooler, leave it: the donor does not need it, he should be sure to leave it in the cooler unopened for recipient. These syringes, which don't have black rubber stoppers or contain latex, are sperm-safe and specifically for artificial insemination.

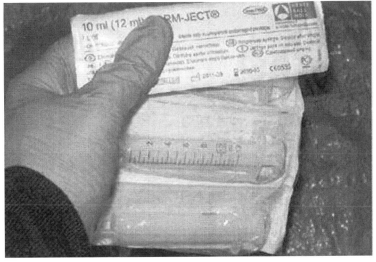

Instead Softcup

The Softcup is a trade name for a type of cervical cap most often used for feminine protection during menstruation (it may have different names, for example "Moon Cup," in different countries). It is also used in artificial insemination as a system for delivering semen into the vagina. If there is an individually wrapped Instead Softcup in the kit, the donor does not need it; he should leave it in the cooler unopened because it is for the recipient to use. I know some donors may be curious, so here is a picture of what it looks like, now you do not need to open it to see!

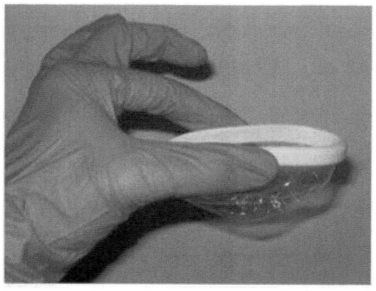

Styrofoam cooler

Place the insulated foil envelope with the vials inside in the bottom of the cooler then place ice packs on top (cold air sinks). (This cooler is purchased from Uline, and comes with the outer cardboard shipping carton mentioned a few pages later; turn to the next chapter for instructions on how to make your own cooler)

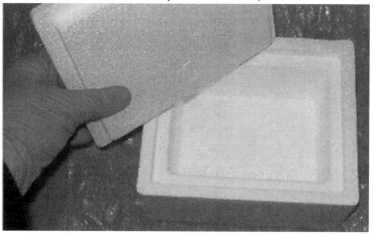

Tape the cooler shut

After placing insulated foil envelope (with semen vials inside), cold pack, and other components in the cooler, seal the lid with tape so cold air will not escape. It is a good idea to keep extra rolls of tape available. They always seem to disappear at the most inopportune time and you will have to buy a $5 roll of tape at the express shipping company.

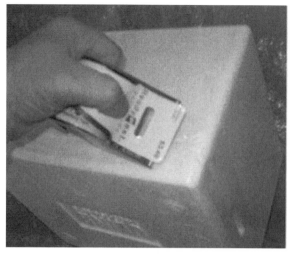

Shipping carton

Place Styrofoam cooler in cardboard shipping carton. Print out the shipping label. For UPS, fold the printout with the label in half and tape to the carton. Be sure to cover the entire label with transparent tape. If shipping with FedEx, they have clear plastic envelopes with adhesive backs; you put the label in it and stick to the package.

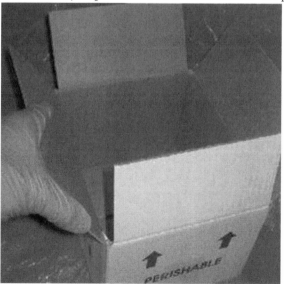

Chapter 15: Solutions for donors who don't have access to a freezer or somewhere to store supplies

Some donors may find themselves without ready access to a refrigerator or freezer when they are trying to ship. For example, they may not want to store their TYB and cold packs in a communal refrigerator where family or friends are storing their food. Some donors may not have anywhere to store Styrofoam boxes bought from Uline or similar vendors. For example, the Uline boxes come in sets of eight, which makes for a very large package, perhaps hard to explain to family members. It would be very difficult for a donor in that situation to ship using traditional, liquid TYB from Irvine in Styrofoam coolers with cold packs purchased from Uline. By using powder extender and shipping kits made from items bought at the supermarket, like cheap thermoses, frozen vegetables, etc., a donor can successfully ship chilled semen much more unobtrusively, since he can avoid mail-order in bulk from companies like Uline, instead buying items as he needs them from the supermarket, and he can also avoid using a refrigerator or freezer. I think the ability to maintain a low profile will appeal to donors who wish to remain anonymous.

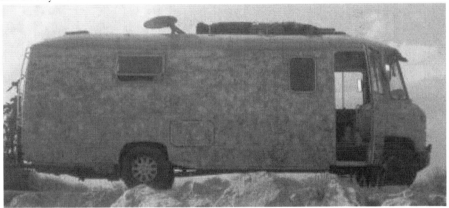

Chapter 16: How to make a homemade Styrofoam cooler

See our YouTube video on how to make a Styrofoam cooler with a utility knife, cardboard box, and sheets of Styrofoam purchased at the hardware store. (http://youtu.be/2qIiKMTCgeU)

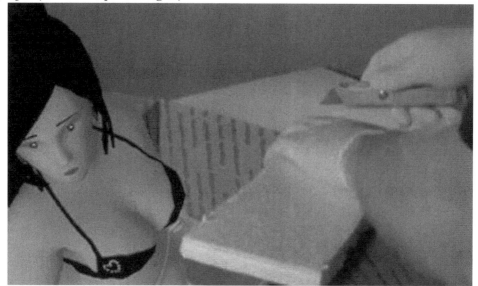

A soldering gun is useful to cut Styrofoam

A knife produces many crumbs of Styrofoam that make a large mess. A soldering gun produces no crumbs and allows you to avoid this mess. You can buy a soldering gun like this one in a hardware store. Maybe it costs $30. This attachable blade is used to cut Styrofoam.

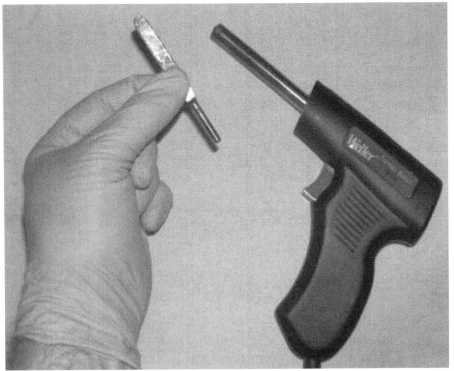

When attaching the blade, be sure that it is aligned with the gun barrel
If the blade is turned sideways, it is harder to cut.

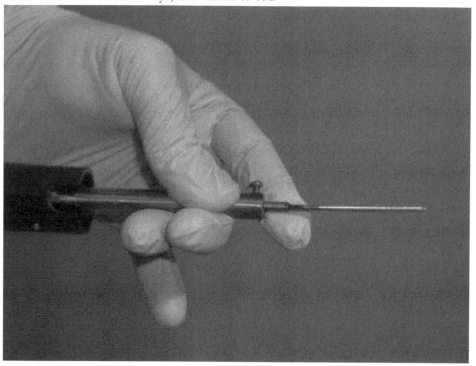

Attach the Styrofoam blade to the soldering gun

Firmly affix the Styrofoam blade to the barrel of the soldering gun using a small screwdriver. Be sure to keep the blade aligned properly.

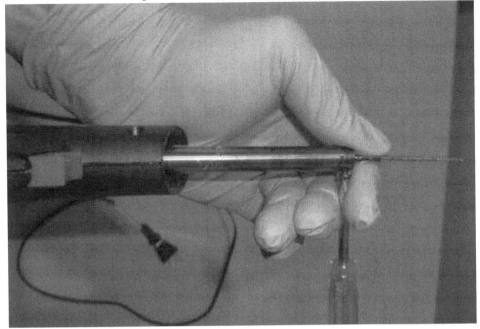

Heat the gun

This model is very simple; it heats automatically when plugged in. The gun has a stand to keep it from burning the surface it is resting on. The gun and the stand are very light. The cord is heavier perhaps than the gun, so it is easy for the cord to drag the gun off a table top. Exercise some caution and be sure the gun is unplugged before leaving the room.

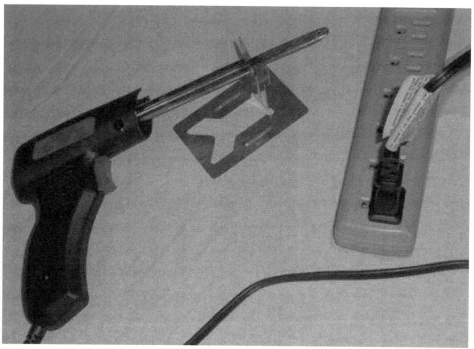

Modify cooler bought in store

I will take this cooler I bought in the supermarket for $3 and modify it.

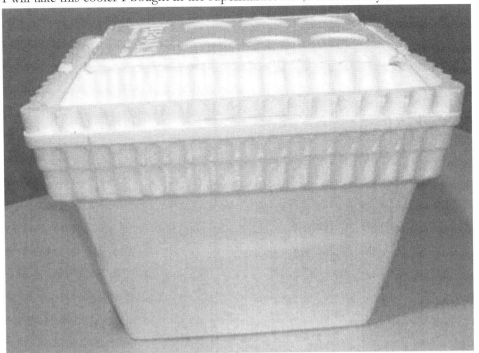

Measure before cutting

I want the modified cooler to fit in this cardboard box that I will use to protect it during shipment. I measure the cooler against the cardboard box. I mark the cooler where I will cut it.

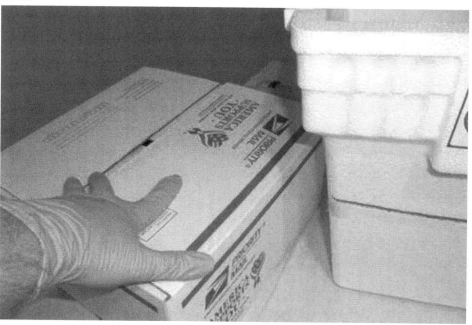

Cut with soldering iron

I cut with the soldering iron. Use a steady hand and don't go to fast. Keep the blade straight, and cut with the upper part of the blade that is closest to the barrel of the gun.

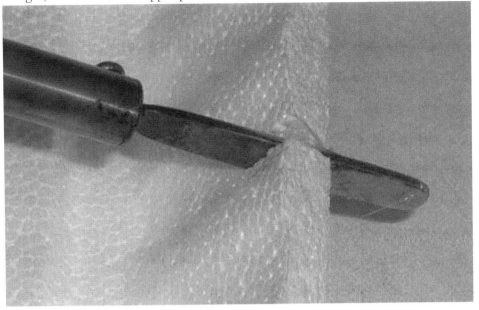

Modify the cardboard box

The box is square. The cooler is rectangular. The box is too short and too wide.

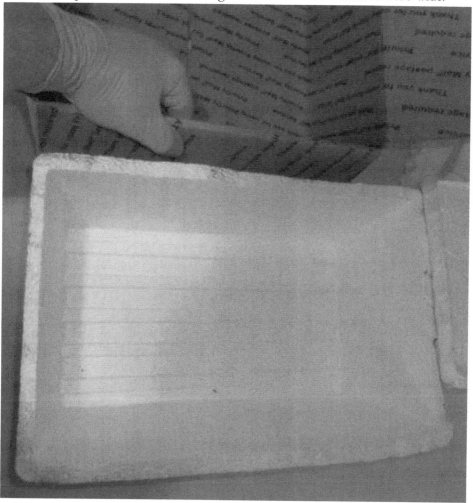

Measure cardboard box and cut

I measure the cardboard box against the Styrofoam cooler. I mark where I will cut it. I cut with a knife.

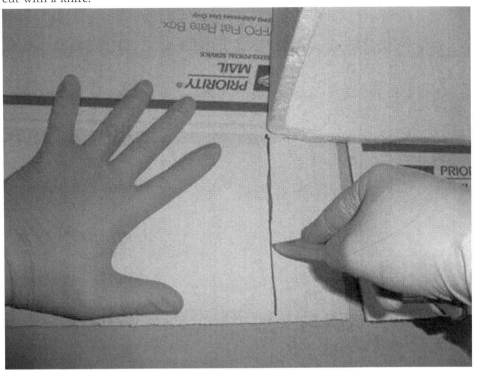

Homemade shipping kit from modified cardboard box and Styrofoam cooler
I tape the box together. I put the modified Styrofoam cooler in it. It is just right.

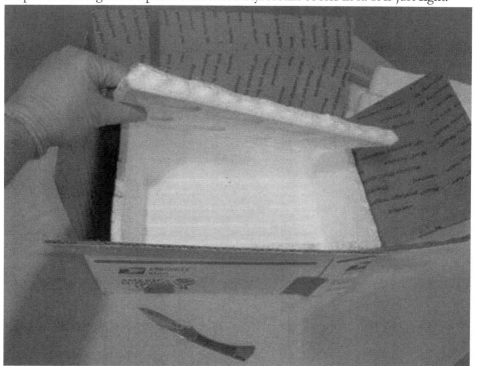

Chapter 17: Shipping chilled semen in a thermos

You can also use a thermos if you cannot find or modify a Styrofoam cooler. This is a very inexpensive thermos purchased for $5. I was in a hurry and didn't have a Styrofoam cooler or cold packs. I purchased the thermos for $5 at the supermarket. Cold air is heavier, so it sinks to the bottom of the container. Put the transport tube with the extended semen at the bottom of the thermos.

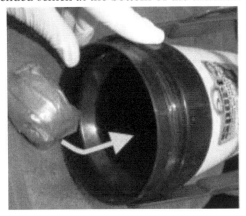
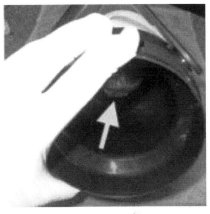

Where to find ready-made coolant?

In this case, I did not have time to freeze cold packs. So, I got some frozen corn at the supermarket. You could of course just buy ice, but typical bags of ice you find at the supermarket are too large, so you would have to carefully repack some of the ice so that it fits in the thermos but doesn't leak, and perhaps discard the left over ice. I think a small bag of frozen vegetables is more convenient. Whichever coolant you use, place it on top of the extended semen.

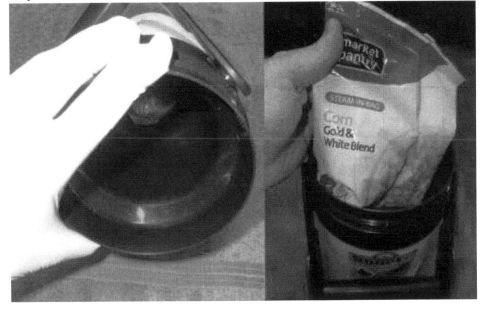

"Reusable ice substitute" as a coolant

These reusable ice substitutes come in bendable sheets. They were in the camping/recreation area at Target, for use in ice chests on picnics. Unlike other coolants, they can be easily rolled up even after they are frozen and fit perfectly in the thermos.

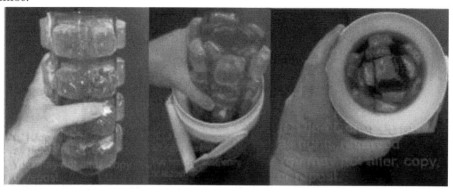

Consider the shape of the coolant when freezing

Consider the form the coolant will take after it is frozen. If, for example, you know the coolant must be flat, or fit in a corner, or be rolled up, be careful to freeze it in the shape it must occupy in the shipping kit. Cardboard is always a convenient material to use to provide forms for coolant to freeze on. Many refrigerators have uneven surfaces on the bottom: in this picture, the floor of the freezer has ridges, so a piece of plastic is used to provide a flat surface for the cold packs to freeze on.

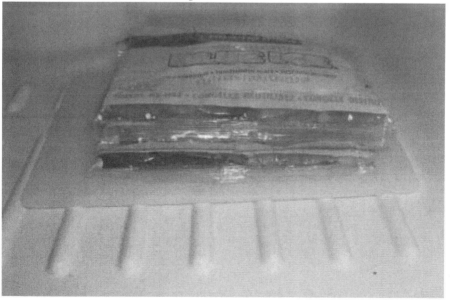

Be sure to consider weather conditions.
In very hot weather, you may need to add additional insulation or additional coolant. This may also increase weight and shipping costs. Those costs should be passed on to the recipient. Especially when shipping in hot weather, there may be a lot of water generated from condensation or leakage from the coolant. Water kills semen. Be sure to carefully pack semen so that the vials aren't exposed to water. For example, carefully tape up the semen in an insulated envelope, or wrap the vials of semen in paper towel and place in a Ziploc bag.

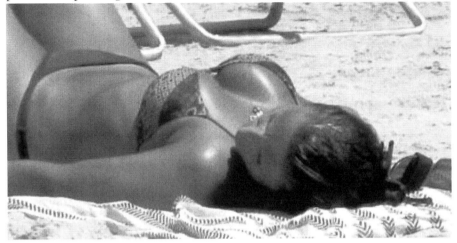

Chapter 18: Drop off at express mail company

Keep aware of locations and hours for your express mail company's local drop off locations so you do not miss the last pick up, or, if you miss it, you know where else may be open later. Know the truck routes. For example, where I live, I know the last pick up for the day is made at the local Armed Forces Recruiting Station. If you have already paid for shipping online and printed out a label, you may be able to give the package to the driver directly. The truck driver won't ask to see your ID, and he tends to ask fewer questions about package contents than the clerks in the company's office.

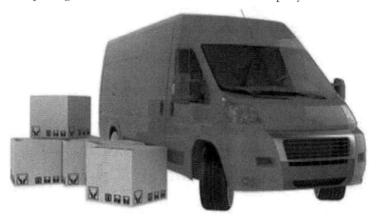

Friday Shipment

You would ship Friday for a positive ovulation test you get on a Friday, possibly also if you expect a positive ovulation test over the weekend. Remember, if you ship overnight on a Friday, you must pay extra. For example, it is an extra $16 for a Saturday deliver when you ship with the U.S. company UPS. With UPS, you must also use a special label for Saturday delivery. If you don't follow the company's rules for Saturday deliveries, the shipment might not arrive until Monday.

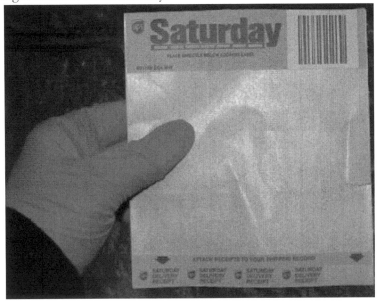

Insure you paid for Saturday delivery and the label has a Saturday code

It usually costs extra for Saturday delivery. I remember once, using the U.S. company UPS, I wasn't charged for a Saturday delivery, and I thought, oh, this is great, I save $16. Unfortunately I was wrong. What actually happens is if you don't pay for Saturday delivery, an "overnight" package that is sent on a Friday arrives on Monday, since that is the next business day. So insure you paid properly and the shipping label has a Saturday code and that there is a visual display for Saturday delivery. This picture is a package shipped on a Friday with the code "1 S" and special orange "Saturday" label for overnight delivery arriving on a Saturday with the U.S. company UPS.

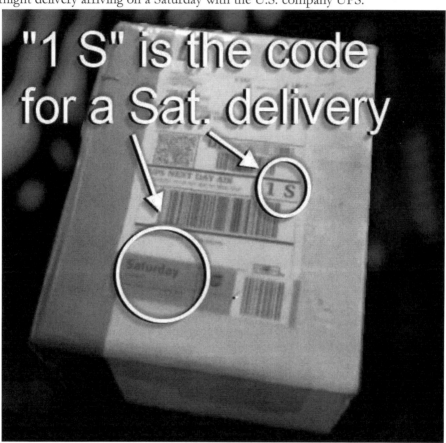

What if the OPK turns positive on a weekend?

Since two out of seven positive opk's will fall on a weekend day, you need to consider your weekend strategy. You need to plan ahead on Friday if you expect a weekend OPK. Since some of the odds are based on whether ovulation comes early or late after the OPK turns positive, and you will never know which it is, shipping multiple days would increase your odds, but also your costs. Since cycle events tend to fall on the same day of the week, week after week, skipping a cycle does not guarantee better timing the next cycle. Skipping a cycle has a zero chance of success: shipping with poor odds may still be better.

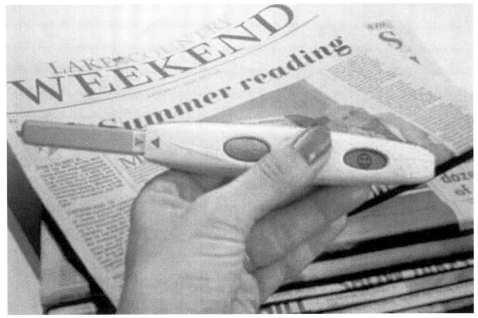

Saturday OPK

Express mail companies are closed on Sunday, so if you get a positive OPK on a Saturday and ship it would not arrive until Monday, by which time the sperm and egg might no longer be viable. You could ship anyway and hope that egg and sperm survive until Monday when the shipment would arrive. Since companies close early on Saturday, you would need to check the OPK early Saturday morning. With the current economic situation, and many businesses cutting back hours, you should call your local express mail services to verify their Saturday availability during the week, do not wait until Saturday. I have microscopically examined sperm kept in the cooler for two days and found some alive, of course this does not mean they would be in ideal shape to fertilize the egg. However, it is possible. You could also ship on Friday if you expect the OPK to turn positive on the weekend, and hope it covers Sunday.

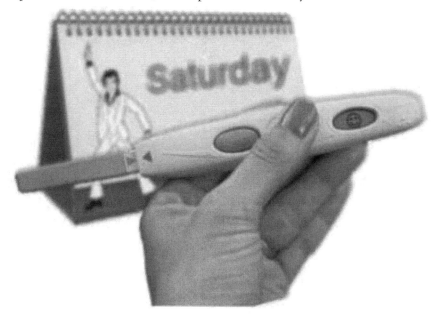

Sunday OPK

Express mail companies are closed on Sunday, so if you get a positive OPK on a Sunday you cannot ship until Monday. You could ship Monday and hope that the egg survives until Tuesday when the shipment would arrive. You could also ship on Saturday if you expect the OPK to turn positive on Sunday and hope that the sperm survive until Monday when the shipment would arrive. I have examined sperm kept in the cooler for two days and found some alive, of course this does not mean they would be in ideal shape to fertilize the egg. However, it is possible. If you already shipped Friday, you could just hope for the best.

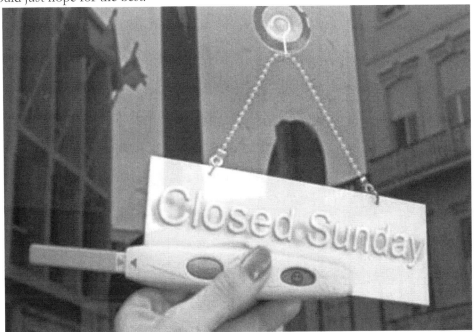

Benefits of holding packages at The UPS Store, other UPS tips

UPS will not deliver to a PO Box, and you will also need a phone number for overnight, although they never call. In a pinch, a donor can use his own phone number if he does not have the recipient's. All my problems with UPS come from delivery truck issues. Consider holding the package at UPS to avoid delivery truck issues. You can have UPS hold the package for pick up by the recipient at a local The UPS Store. If held at a local The UPS Store it may also arrive sooner than residential deliveries, and does not spend all day bouncing around in the back of a hot truck. In some rural areas, next day residential delivery is not possible: instead deliver to a nearby The UPS Store.

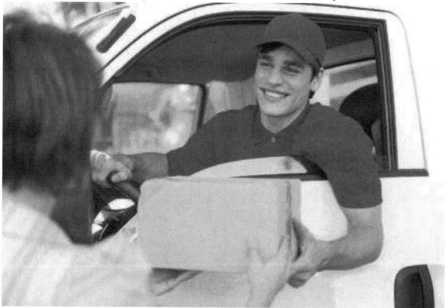

Benefits of holding packages at the express mail company's office and other tips

In the USA, UPS will not deliver to a post office box, and we must provide a phone number for overnight shipping. Other express mail companies around the world may have similar requirements. If I do not know the recipient's phone number, I can write in any number I like, for example, my own number, and they accept the package. If there is no problem with delivery, they never call. However, if there is a delivery problem, for example they cannot find the address, they may call, and if the recipient hasn't provided a number, or someone else's number was used, she may not be able direct the truck to her address. All my problems in the USA with UPS come from delivery truck issues. Here in the USA, UPS has local franchise stores, called "The UPS Store,", and they will hold a package for free until the recipient picks it up. This is a great option if a recipient wants to protect her privacy and not provide her home address and phone number. If the package is held at the local office, it may also arrive sooner than it would if it is sent out for residential delivery. In very warm weather, the package may sit in the back of a hot truck all day while waiting for residential delivery, which may overcome the insulation and cold pack and cause the shipped sample to heat up, adversely affecting sperm quality. Holding the package at the local store allows you to avoid the package overheating in the back of a truck in warm weather. In some rural areas, next day residential delivery is not possible, but the package can be delivered to a local office that is not too far away. So be sure to learn about your options with local offices of the express mail company that you use. **Although shipping companies which hold packages for pick up may ask the recipient for ID, in practice, they usually do not.**

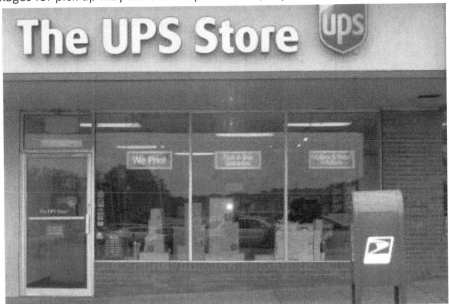

UPS Customer Centers

Express mail companies often have central or regional collection facilities where they load and unload large trucks to transfer to smaller trucks for local delivery. The central/regional offices may be open later than the local offices. Learn if the company you use has such a center in case you miss the last local pick up. In my case, I use UPS in the USA, the regional office, or "Customer Service Center," is 30 minutes away from me by car, but it is open until 9pm while the local office closes at 5pm. If I miss the 5pm closing, I can still drop off at 9pm, although I have to drive another 30 minutes, I won't miss the shipment. Find out if the company you use has a central collection facility near your recipient. In the USA, I use UPS, and I can have UPS hold the package for pick up by the recipient at a Customer Center. If it is held at the Customer Center, the recipient can pick it up at 9am in morning when the Customer Center opens. In the USA, UPS offers an early morning home delivery, for an extra fee. But she can pick it up at 9am at the Customer Center, earlier than the earliest residential delivery, and there is no fee.

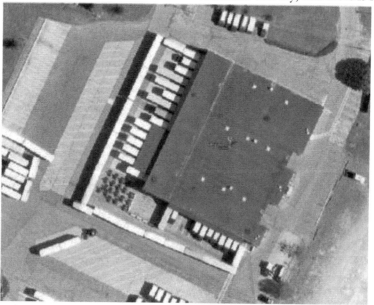

Express mail companies may ask for ID

Express mail companies may ask for ID, at the pick up or at drop off. This might cause concern for donors who wish to remain anonymous. If the donor pays for shipping and fill out paper work at the drop off location, he may need to show ID. However, if the donor pays and prints out a shipping label at home, he may be able to drop off the package with the clerk at the drop off location without showing ID. If the donor pays online and prints out the label at home, he can also give the package to the driver directly, and the drivers never ask for ID.

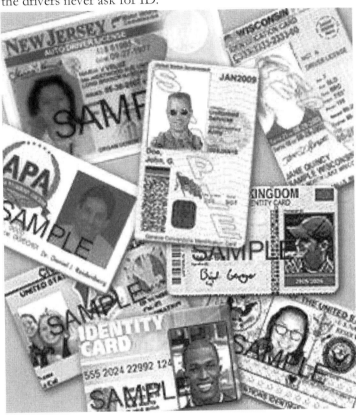

Drop off boxes

Some companies will have drop off boxes that are unmanned. Be sure to check the size of the opening to the drop off box to make sure your package will fit in it. Also be sure to check the last pick up time. This is usually written on the drop off box. I prefer to leave the package with a person, but if it fits in the drop box, that should also work. Try also to use a drop box that is not in direct sunlight, or avoid leaving the package too soon before the last pick up if it is extremely hot or cold outside.

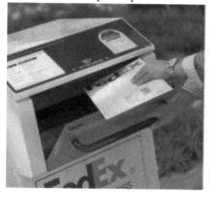
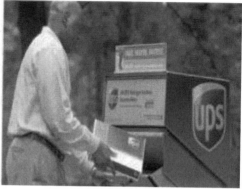

Early morning delivery

In the USA, UPS offers an early morning home delivery, for an extra fee. But a recipient can also pick it up at 9am at the Customer Center, earlier than the earliest residential delivery, and there is no fee. This may be a better option if there is a Customer Center nearby. Even if you are not using UPS, other express delivery services may have similar options, so you should investigate well before the big day arrives. (I use UPS in the USA, and UPS calls their regional central collection centers, where they collect packages for bulk shipping, "Customer Service Centers," if you are outside the USA, or use a different company in the USA, they probably have a similar organization, but you would need to check with them to see what they call their regional collection centers and what are the hours, locations, and other details for those centers.)

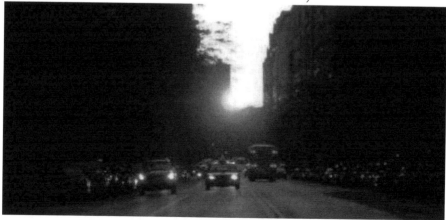

Chapter 19: For recipients: Basic insemination with syringe

Do not keep part to use later. Recipients should inseminate with all the semen as soon as the package arrives. Some women erroneously think keeping part of the contents in the refrigerator means they can do a second insemination a day later and increase their odds. Do not do this, it will lower your chances, sperm survives, longer in the female reproductive track than anywhere else, and you need a certain volume to get pregnant. Since some die in shipping, everyone that is left needs to get inside. Special thanks to Eric Donor (Ej2004/Spudster2010) for the image, which is of an anatomically correct model and not a real vagina.

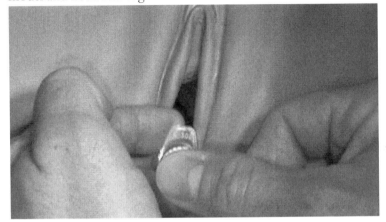

Macroscopic examination of the semen (how the semen should appear to the naked eye)

Fresh semen is normally more transparent, and off white, but chilled shipped semen may be more yellowish in color and opaque, due to the addition of TYB, which has yellow egg yolk in it. Semen may have bubbles. This is perfectly normal. It may smell strongly, like Clorox. Volume of the chilled sample will be anywhere from 5-10ml typically, since the normal ejaculate volume ranges from 2.5-5ml, plus an equal volume of extender is added. The recipient may notice some sediment in the extended semen (that is, there may appear to be particles resting at the bottom of the transport tube). This is normal, as the sperm are not moving, and may clump together and sink to the bottom, or some of the extender may precipitate out of solution. Just gently shake to mix it again before insemination.

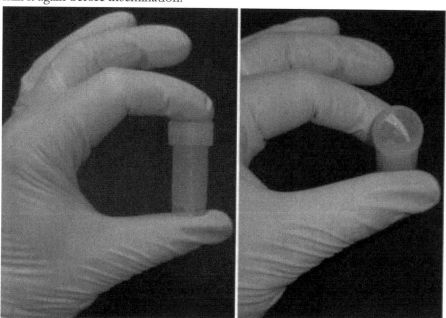

For some reason many women expect more volume

For some reason many women expect more volume, perhaps it is due to the abnormal amounts of ejaculate that are often depicted in pornography. It is worth noting that in pornography many tricks are used, such as splicing in several clips of the same ejaculation taken from different angles, or even fake semen, to make the volume seem larger. In reality, 5ml (10ml with extender) is a large sample, and 2.5ml (5ml with extender) is still in the normal range. Still, the more volume the greater the chance of success, so a donor who consistently provides samples in the upper normal range is preferable, although anyone can experience variation in volume without it impacting fertility. The picture is fresh semen (without extender added) so you must imagine a volume of twice as much in the case of chilled semen with extender.

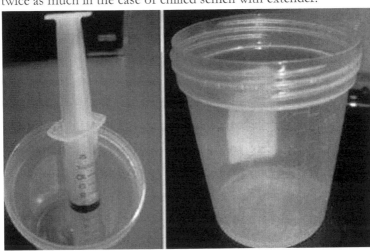

Sterile, individually wrapped, 10ml syringe

The recipient inseminates with the included 10ml syringe (specifically designed for artificial insemination, no black rubber or latex). If there is no syringe in the cooler, you can buy one at CVS, Wal-Mart, Walgreens, etc. If you do not see it in the aisle, ask at the pharmacy. Shy? Say you need it to give cough syrup to your baby since it won't use the cup included with the cough syrup. They often times have them for free in the pharmacy if they are not on sale on the floor. Before you ovulate, you should inform yourself of where these stores are located, their hours, and if they have the supplies you need. Do not wait until the last minute.

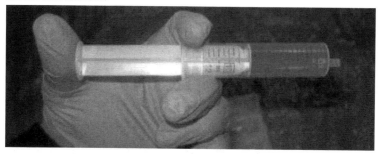

If vial mouth is too small, pour semen in cup

If vial mouths are too small for the syringe to fit in to aspirate the contents, pour contents in to a sterile specimen cup or clean glass. If using a glass, wash and rinse well with hot water: make sure any soap is rinsed out of the glass, soap residue can cause more harm than whatever substance was cleaned out of glass. You could also use an extension on the end of the syringe, such as a blunt, 18-gauge needle, etc. With care it is possible to pull the plunger out of the syringe and pour the semen in the back, but I think aspirating from the front is safer. If you can find a short sterile tube or cut a piece with scissors from a longer sterile tube or hose that is the right circumference, fit it firmly to the syringe, and aspirate that way.

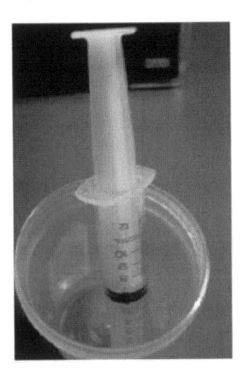

Insemination with 10ml syringe (needle-less)

Insert syringe in to vagina. The contents of the syringe should be injected in to the vagina steadily. If the plastic syringe sticks, and too much force is applied too quickly, the syringe plunger could slip, break, pop out, etc. Applying a small amount of a sperm safe lubricant to the plunger beforehand may avoid sticking. Some recommend that the recipient masturbate herself in order to induce an orgasm at the time of insemination in order to draw the semen in to the cervix. It is also recommended that she lay supine for at least 10 minutes after insem with hips raised so that the semen will not run out.

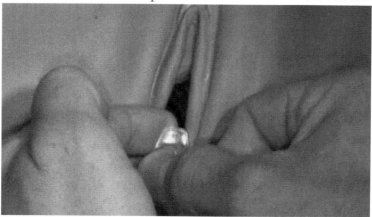

Chapter 20: Insemination using speculum and catheter

Insertion of speculum: Insert with the bills closed and vertical in regard to the vaginal orifice. Once inside, rotate until the bills are horizontal in regard to the vagina, and open. If a lubricant is necessary, be sure to use one that is sperm-friendly. Special thanks to Ej2004/Spudster2010 for the images, which are of an anatomically correct model and not a real vagina.

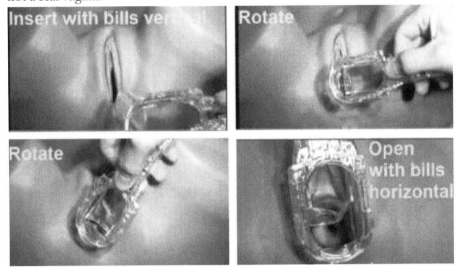

Catheter detail

Aspirate semen into syringe, attach catheter, insert into open speculum, and advance catheter near to cervix (do not enter in to the cervix, the cervix filters everything but sperm out of the semen; introduction of raw semen in to the uterus could cause violent uterine contractions). Confirm catheter tip location, and depress plunger. Remove syringe and speculum. Some recommend that the recipient masturbate herself in order to induce an orgasm at the time of insemination in order to draw the semen in to the cervix. It is also recommended that she lay supine for at least 10 minutes after insem with hips raised so that the semen will not run out.

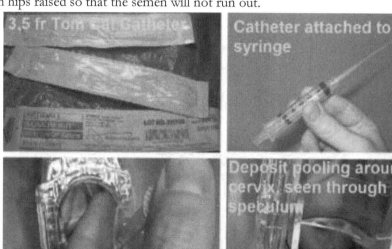
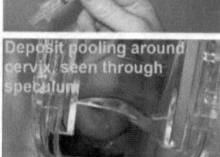

Chapter 21: Instead Softcup insemination

"Softcup" is a trade name for a cervical cap used in the USA for feminine protection during menstruation. In other countries, it may have a different name. The vials of extended semen can be poured in to a Softcup for insertion into the vagina instead of using a syringe. The Softcup, as a new fad, seems to be popular, however, I see no reason why it should be better than a syringe, and no one has compared the efficacy of the two for achieving pregnancy in a scientific study. Some kits include a Softcup, if yours does not, you can also buy one at CVS, Wal-Mart, Walgreens, etc. Since they are easy to obtain, they could be used in lieu of a syringe if you cannot obtain a syringe. Before you ovulate, you should inform yourself of where you may obtain syringes, Softcups, etc., store hours, and the like. Do not wait until the last minute. Some recommend that the recipient masturbate herself in order to induce an orgasm at the time of insemination with the Softcup in order to draw the semen in to the cervix. It is also recommended that she lay supine for at least 10 minutes after insem with hips raised so that the semen will not run out. Unless you are using the Softcup in lieu of a syringe, I don't think it is necessary to insert a Softcup for the sole purpose of preventing semen from running out, I believe that most sperm that is going to swim up the female reproductive tract does so soon after insemination, and the semen that runs out isn't affecting a woman's chances to get pregnant. Do not leave a Softcup in for more than 12 hours. I believe that 1-2 hours is probably more than long enough.

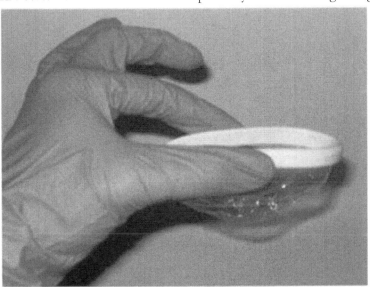

How to insert the Softcup

Pinch the Softcup into a figure eight as shown in the picture. Sometimes it helps to put lubricant on the leading edge of the Softcup. If lubricant is necessary, use one that is sperm-safe. Keeping the Softcup pressed in to a figure eight shape, push it completely into the vagina. Using your finger, push it down and back as far as it will go. It will slip into place under the cervix and behind the pubic bone. I helped a recipient a few times doing this, even the first time it was very easy to do, although I had never done it before. I think it is much better for the recipient to lay back and have someone else insert the Softcup even though she could do it herself. The recipient and whoever is helping her may want to practice before the insemination so they do not risk spilling the semen.

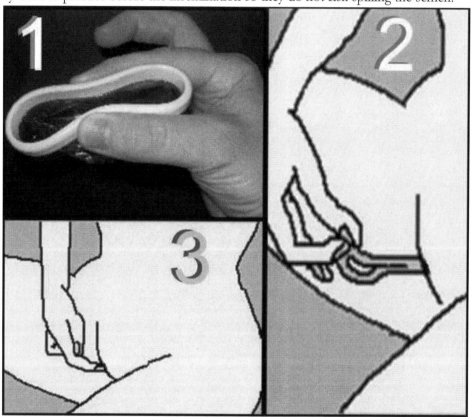

Chapter 22: What about the turkey baster?

The turkey baster is famous for being used in attempted artificial insemination in the American TV. drama "Brookside." It is actually quite clumsy to use in comparison with a 10ml syringe. As you can see, the bore of the mouth is much larger, volume is much larger, and it does not efficiently produce a vacuum in comparison with the syringe. It is simply too large an instrument for semen and might work, but might also deposit your sample accidentally on your bed sheet, couch, car seat, or wherever you are when you inseminate.

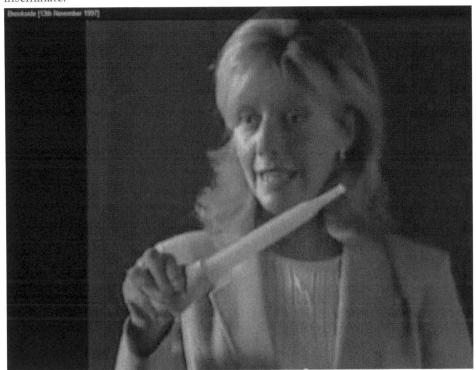

(Brookside episode of November 13, 1997, http://youtu.be/BUzywFJie0U)

The turkey is a large bird that is traditionally eaten on some holidays in the U.S.

For readers who are not from the USA and who may be unfamiliar with the turkey baster, basting is a cooking technique in which meat is cooked in a marinade or in its own juices. The liquid that runs off the meat and collects in the pan is periodically scooped up using the baster, a syringe like instrument, and reapplied to the meat. The turkey is a large bird that is traditionally eaten on some holidays in the U.S. It dries out easily, so basting is necessary, and most homes have a turkey baster on hand, even though they probably wouldn't have a syringe lying around.

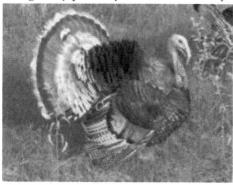
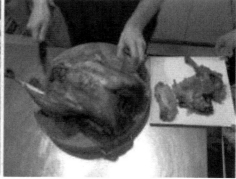

The turkey baster is clumsy to use in comparison with a 10ml syringe

The turkey baster is the mascot of lesbian artificial insemination and a hero of legend. However, they are quite clumsy to use in comparison with a 10ml syringe. As you can see, the bore of the mouth is much larger, volume is much larger, and it does not efficiently produce a vacuum in comparison with the syringe. It is simply too large an instrument for semen and might work, but might also deposit your sample accidentally on your bed sheet, couch, car seat, or wherever you are when you inseminate.

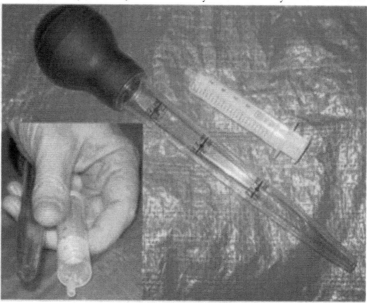

Chapter 23: Check shipped sperm microscopically to see if still alive

A macroscopic examination will not show you if the sperm is alive, but microscope can be used to check. Here is a video screen shot from a Lab Clinic Trinocular Microscope from amscope.com. In live video, you can see many sperm moving. A Live-Dead stain has been used to show which are alive (hollow circles are live sperm). It is a fairly expensive set up, very technical, using not only an oil lens on the microscope but also toxic Live-Dead stain that must also be shipped chilled. It might be easier to choose a donor who is already set up for checking sperm with a microscope. He can keep a small portion of your sample in an extra shipping kit and test it when he sees from tracking that your shipment has arrived.

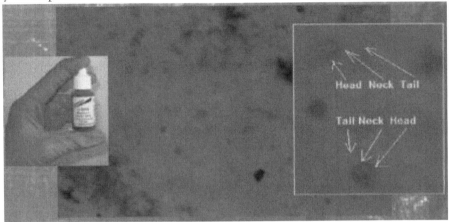

Micra Hand-held scope specifically for the evaluation of sperm

This is a simpler and less expensive set up. It is only 200x magnification but simpler to use. It can still be a little tricky to catch the sperm on a microscope. Since it is a thick liquid, if you are not searching on the right plane you could miss it think the sample is void of sperm. You must focus carefully until you find the sperm. You must also keep in mind that the sample is diluted with an equal volume of extender, throwing off sperm counts. The slide should be warmed to body temperature; otherwise the sperm may appear to have poor motility.

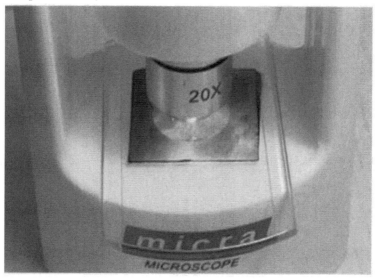

Prepare a semen smear slide

1. Use a sterile pipette to collect a small amount of semen from the container the donor used for collection. You could also collect some that has run out after insemination. Drop a very small droplet slightly off-center on the slide. (If the drop is too large, you can use another coverslip to transfer part of it to a new slide). 2. Holding the edges of the slide edge that is furthest from the droplet between thumb and index finger of your left hand, take a coverslip in the fingers of your right hand, so that you pinch the top between your thumb and index finger and the coverslip is tilted to the right at an angle of between 30-40 degrees from the slide. 3. Slowly move it toward the semen until it contacts the leading edge and "grabs" the droplet. 4. Without changing the tilt of the coverslip, move it back toward your left over the slide, so as to drag the semen across the slide creating a smear. Once you are slightly past the center and before the smear is longer than the coverslip, gently let the coverslip fall back on the smear.

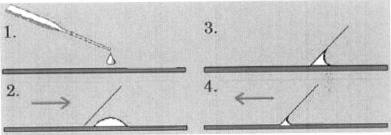

Use a donor who knows how to evaluate sperm microscopically

Recipients can buy a scope and evaluate the shipped sample themselves. However, they are unlikely to get enough experience to become proficient at this, and may not want to spend the extra money. A popular shipping donor quickly becomes experienced at microscopic evaluation. He can keep a small amount of the shipped sample and place it in another cooler at the same time he packages the main sample for the recipient. He can see from the tracking what time it arrives, and evaluate his sample soon after the recipient receives hers. As you can see, quite possible to take pictures even video with a digital camera through the hand-held scope. Teaching sperm analysis is beyond the scope of this book, but the more experienced donors know how to do this already, and this type of experience might be a criterion recipients want to consider when choosing a donor.

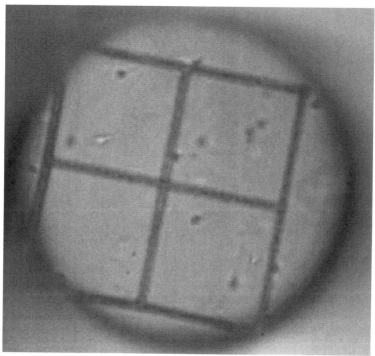

Chapter 24: When can I do the HPT (home pregnancy test)?

Congratulations, you have done all you can, now it is up to the sperm and egg. Depending on the hpt (home pregnancy test) brand, you can test starting as early as 10dpo (days past ovulation). Chances of a false negative are less if you can wait till 14dpo. Remember, unlike the OPK, a faint line on the HPT IS positive (all the below tests were positive). Be sure to inform your donor of the results, so he can share in the joy, or prepare for the next donation.

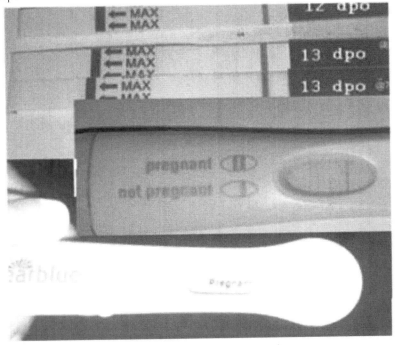

Unusual pregnancy test results

Can you get a positive and a negative pregnancy test in the same day?

In this case, the positive is from first urine of the morning. Hcg is concentrated overnight that is why first urine is best for the hpt. The negative is from second urine, hcg is more diluted. This is only 11 or 12dpo, so the hcg is only at the threshold for the test probably and the difference in hcg in first and second urine of the morning was enough to cause a false negative.

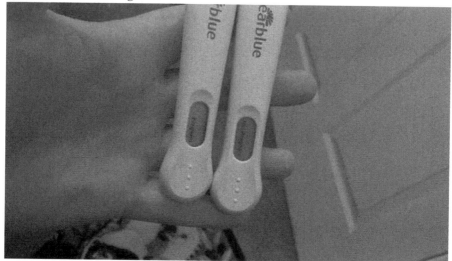

A faint test line is a positive on the HPT

A very fine test line was later obtained on a different test. Again, a faint positive is always a positive with the hpt, and one needs to be aware of differences in brands.

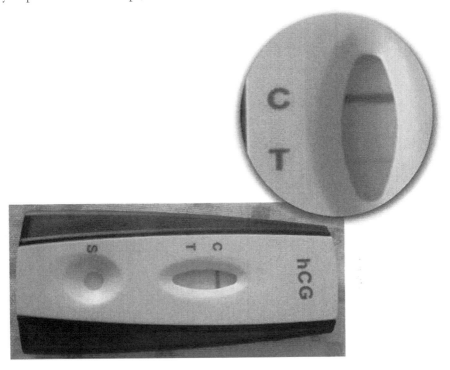

Chapter 25: How far away can I ship?

Technology is always improving. Styrofoam and cold packs allow us to ship almost anywhere in a large country such as the USA within 12-36 hours. Sperm has a useful life of about 24-48 hours, so this timeframe allows success, but success rates improve if delivery can be faster. Early morning delivery and late night drop off can reduce this to about 12 hours for destinations that are close by. For example, if you can drop off at 8pm, as we can at a UPS Service Center in the USA for example, and have a 9am pick up by the recipient at a UPS Service Center near her, it is possible, but often time's donor and recipient won't have a Service Center that is nearby. A 24-hour turn around, with a 4pm drop off and 4pm delivery the next day, is more normal.

Delivery companies like Amazon are now experimenting with drones. One day, drones and other new technologies may allow shipped semen to arrive even more quickly.

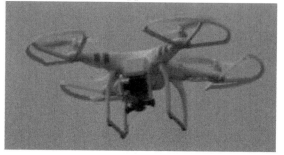

However, even though technology improves, new legal restrictions cause delays. Delays at customs make international shipping difficult if not possible between most countries.

We know shipping from Canada to the USA is done easily, while shipping from the USA to Canada is difficult. I do not personally know of international shipping successes aside from the Canada to USA route.

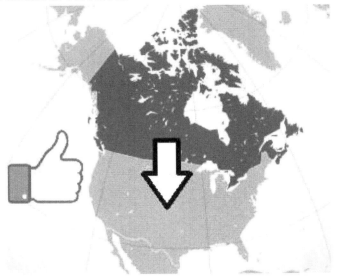

International shipping from Germany to France and from Germany to the UK

I have heard rumors of shipping between Germany and the UK, or Germany and France, and I think this would be possible and might succeed, I don't know for sure. As long as overnight delivery is available, it should be possible to achieve pregnancy. It is still an area that needs more exploration.

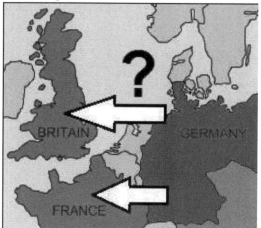

Shipping from the USA to Scotland?

I have heard of shipping from the USA to Scotland, but it takes 48 hours at least, and I doubt this could succeed. Due to the youth of the chilled semen shipping industry, and the difficulty of obtaining traditional semen extenders, such as Irvine's TYB, which must be kept frozen and are often controlled by laboratories, there is little information on shipping within Europe and other locations. Hopefully this will change with the new powder extenders described in this book, which don't need to be refrigerated until they are prepared for use. In the future more countries may control the shipment of semen for public health reasons, or place restrictions on private donors, although these laws seem difficult to enforce at the present. So, we recommend you should start shipping as soon as possible if this is something that you want to do.

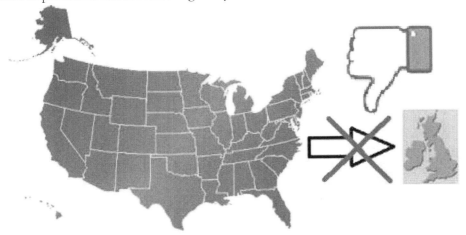

Chapter 26: Use a chemical heating and cooling pack to prevent freezing in extreme cold

In cold climates, the semen may freeze. Freezing will kill the sperm. You can use a chemical heating and cooling pack to control the temperature. The pack has a chemical in it that changes to liquid/solid at 60 or 70 degrees Fahrenheit. If the temperature exceeds 60-70 degrees F, it changes to liquid, and absorbs energy from the surroundings, causing cooling. It the temperature falls below 60-70 degrees, it changes to solid, releasing energy, and this causes heating. You can put a cold pack right next to the sample to keep it cool in an inner container. Then, you put the heating and cooling pack in the outer box, separated by insulation from the sample and cold pack, so that it controls temperature extremes.

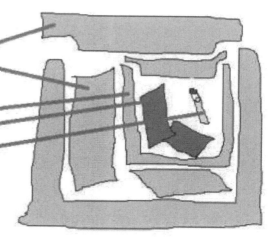

1. **Outer container**
2. **Heating/cooling pack**
3. **Inner container**
4. **Cold pack**
5. **Sample**

Chapter 27: Testing a prototype of shipping kit

Once you make a shipping container prototype, you must test it under the weather conditions in which you expect to use it: Spring and fall are often very forgiving, while summer in warmer latitudes, and winter in colder latitudes, can present challenges. In this example, a specimen cup with water has been placed in the cooler with cold packs. A hole was bored through the cooler and the top of the specimen cup. A thermometer was inserted through the holes to measure the changes in the water temperature. It is also possible to keep a prototype at home, and when you ship to the recipient, keep a small amount of the sample inside your prototype. You can monitor temperatures, and then, when the sample arrives at the recipient's place (you will know when it arrives from the tracking number) you can remove the small amount that you kept and view it with the microscope to see if the sperm are still motile. Remember, you must warm the slide to body temperature before viewing, or the sperm will not move due to the cold.

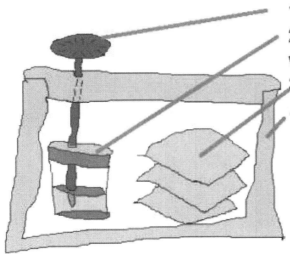

1. **Thermometer**
2. **Specimen cup w/water**
3. **Cold packs**
4. **Container**

This concludes our presentation. Good luck with your TTC efforts!
THE END

If you enjoyed this book, we hope you will enjoy some other titles by Joe Donor (continue to next page for list of some other titles). Please be sure to leave a review on the book's web site and see other titles by Joe Donor:
https://www.smashwords.com/profile/view/joe00donor

Other books by Joe Donor

"Get Pregnant For Free on the Internet With a Private Sperm Donor Without Having Sex or Paying $$$ to a Sperm Bank"
Print version www.createspace.com/4712907
Google ISBN 1497327253 to find where to by the print version if you are not in the USA.
For ebook, Google ASIN B00GGR5I62.
Email Joe Donor at joe00donor@gmail.com to purchase directly.

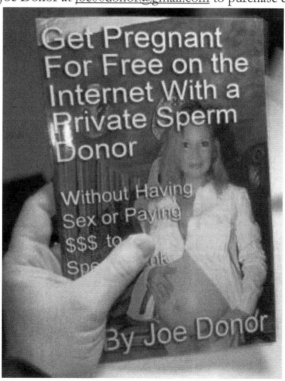

(Continue to next page for more books by Joe Donor) ==>

"True Stories of Pregnancy by PI, or Partial Intercourse, With Free Sperm Donors"

Print version: https://www.createspace.com/4704542
For other places to buy the print version, Google ISBN 1496171977.
Ebook: https://www.smashwords.com/books/view/415423
For other places to buy the ebook version, Google ASIN B00ISCN4ZK
Email Joe Donor at joe00donor@gmail.com to purchase directly.

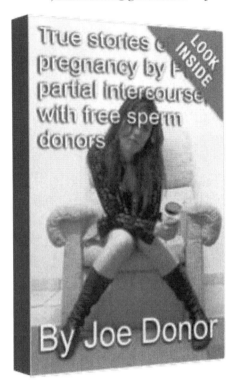

Printed in Poland
by Amazon Fulfillment
Poland Sp. z o.o., Wrocław